HANDBOOK OF CLINICAL PREVENTION

HANDBOOK OF CLINICAL PREVENTION

EDITED BY

Hannelore F. Vanderschmidt, Ph.D.
Associate Professor of Education
Co-Director
Center for Educational Development in Health
Boston University
Visiting Lecturer
Department Health Policy and Management
Harvard School of Public Health
Boston, Massachusetts

Dieter K. Koch-Weser, M.D., Ph.D.
Former Associate Dean and Chairman
Department of Preventive and Social Medicine
Harvard Medical School
Boston, Massachusetts

Patricia A. Woodbury, C.R.N., M.S.N., C.P.N.A.
Health Consultant
Fellow and Member of the National Association of Pediatric Nurse Associates and
    Practitioners
Apple Valley, Minnesota

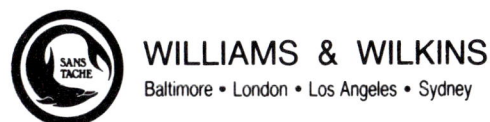

WILLIAMS & WILKINS
Baltimore • London • Los Angeles • Sydney

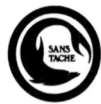

Editor: Nancy Collins
Associate Editor: Carol Eckhart
Design: JoAnne Janowiak
Illustration Planning: Wayne Hubbel
Production: Anne G. Seitz

Copyright © 1987
Williams & Wilkins
428 East Preston Street
Baltimore, MD 21202, U.S.A.

All rights reserved. This book is protected by copyright. No part of this book may be reproduced in any form or by any means, including photocopying, or utilized by any information storage and retrieval system without written permission from the copyright owner.

Printed in the United States of America

Library of Congress Cataloging in Publication Data

Handbook of clinical prevention.

   Includes index.
   1. Medicine, Preventive—Handbooks, manuals, etc. 2. Medicine, Clinical—Handbooks, manuals, etc. I. Vanderschmidt, Hannelore F. II. Koch-Weser, Dieter K. III. Woodbury, Patricia A. [DNLM: 1. Preventive Medicine—handbooks. WA 39 H2353]
RA427.2.H36 1987   613   86-19089
ISBN 0-683-08578-6

Foreword
Ascher J. Segall, M.D., Dr. P.H.

Historically, the education of health practitioners in preventive medicine has been responsive to changes in the patterns of disease, progress in health technology, and shifts in societal priorities. In the early decades of the 20th century, the foremost health problems in the United States were still those of infectious diseases. Rapid scientific advances opened the way for the development of effective preventive measures. Certain interventions, such as immunizations, could be implemented in clinical settings. Others, such as sanitary control, called for action at the community level. A dual role was expected of physicians and nurses; providing preventive care within the context of clinical practice and participating in the community-based public health activities. There was little ambiguity concerning the scope of the subject matter to be learned and the skills to be acquired. Both were derived directly from the responsibilities which students would assume in their future roles within the health care system.

The situation changed significantly as the prevalence of epidemic diseases receded. Atherosclerosis, cancer and other chronic conditions emerged as major causes of disability and death. Etiology, for the most part, was poorly understood and few methods for early detection were known. Under these circumstances, there was little the practicing physician or nurse could do to prevent the onset of these conditions or decrease their rate of progression. An effective role for practitioners in clinical prevention was clearly contingent on a better understanding of the pertinent risk factors and their distribution in the population, the availability of appropriate screening procedures, and more effective measures for primary and secondary prevention.

Reflecting these developments, the emphasis in teaching preventive medicine shifted from clinical applications to the population-oriented disciplines of epidemiology, biostatistics, medical sociology and health care delivery. Only through extensive research in these fields could the knowledge needed for prevention of chronic diseases be generated. In the interim, however, the congruence between curriculum and professional practice evident in the earlier era of infectious diseases was increasingly called into question. The gap between content of instruction and the needs of practicing clinicians continued to widen.

In recent years, the situation has come full circle. Research is indeed beginning to yield new and potentially more effective approaches to health maintenance. Some have clinical applications and can be integrated into practice settings. This has led to a resurgence of interest in the knowledge and skills needed for clinical health maintenance and attitudes which facilitate the process. To the extent that these can be clearly indentified and effectively communicated, the gap between what students learn and what they will need for future professional practice can be bridged.

Bridging the gap is the purpose of a project for curriculum development in clinical prevention initiated about a decade ago by the Center for Educational Development in Health at Boston University and the Association of Teachers of Preventive Medicine. I had the privilege of directing the first six years of the project. A competency-based approach was adopted to reflect the capabilities needed by practitioners in clinical settings. The starting point was a study of current performance patterns in clinical prevention. Three areas of performance emerged as warranting special attention; managing a practice-based program of clinical prevention, determining health and risk status, and assisting patients in modification of behavior patterns.

To facilitate acquisition of these capabilities, a comprehensive instructional system was developed. It was designed by a panel of epidemiologists, primary care providers and medical specialists, in close collaboration with behavioral scientists and educational technologists. The system comprises a set of competency-based learning objectives and a series of corresponding instructional modules. These provide guidance for student learning in academic settings, as well as for the introduction of preventive initiatives in primary care practices. After several years of field-testing and revision, the system is being used in schools of medicine and nursing as well as in programs of continuing education across the United States.

This volume is a distillate of the larger work. It appears in response to a growing demand on the part of students, teachers and practitioners for a practical and concise guide to clinical health maintenance. The frame of reference is the same set of practice-related competencies treated more extensively in the instructional modules. For many readers, the level of detail will suffice. Others may wish to pursue certain topics in further depth by consulting the appropriate modules or other of the references provided.

"Health for all" has been designated by the World Health Organization as a goal to be pursued in all countries. Health, in that context, is viewed as a means of achieving a social and economically productive life which implies far more than just the absence of disease. Rather, it calls for a wide range of proactive and promotive efforts so that people can develop to their full potential. This book can contribute to attaining the WHO goal by narrowing the gap between learning and practice in clinical health maintenance. I therefore hope that it will be widely used by undergraduate and graduate students in the health professions, as well as in the continuing education of health care providers.

> Ascher J. Segall, M.D., Dr.P.H.
> Geneva, Switzerland
> August 1986

Contributors

William H. Barker, Jr., M.D.
Associate Professor
Department of Preventive, Family and Rehabilitation Medicine
University of Rochester
School of Medicine and Dentistry
Rochester, New York

Robert C. Benfari, Ph.D.
Lecturer in Psychology
Harvard School of Public Health
Boston, Massachusetts

Dieter Koch-Weser, M.D., Ph.D.
Former Associate Dean and Chairman
Department of Preventive and Social Medicine
Harvard Medical School
Boston, Massachusetts

Victoria Logan Lamberton, B.A.
Senior Research Associate
Center for Educational Development in Health
Boston University
Boston, Massachusetts

Ascher J. Segall, M.D., Dr.P.H.
Chief Medical Officer
Health Manpower Research
World Health Organization
Geneva, Switzerland

Joseph Stokes III, M.D.
Professor of Medicine and Public Health
Section of Preventive Medicine and Epidemiology
Boston University School of Medicine
Boston, Massachusetts

G. Frederick Vanderschmidt, Ph.D.
Management Consultant
Adjunct Faculty
School of Management
University of Massachusetts
Boston, Massachusetts

Hannelore F. Vanderschmidt, Ph.D.
Associate Professor of Education
Co-Director
Center for Educational Development in Health
Boston University
Visiting Lecturer on Health Policy and Management
Harvard School of Public Health
Boston, Massachusetts

Patricia A. Woodbury, C.R.N., M.S.N., C.P.N.A.
Health Consultant
Fellow and Member of the National Association of Pediatric Nurse
  Associates and Practitioners
Apple Valley, Minnesota

Contents

		Page
Foreword...		v
Ascher J. Segall, M.D., Dr.P.H.		
Acknowledgements...		ix
Contributors...		xi
Chapter 1.	Introduction: The Place of the Practice of Clinical Prevention in Health Care............... Dieter Koch-Weser, M.D., Ph.D.	1
Chapter 2.	The Epidemiologic Basis of Clinical Prevention.... William H. Barker, Jr., M.D.	5
Chapter 3.	The Methods of Clinical Prevention................ Joseph Stokes III, M.D.	29
Chapter 4.	Preventive Initiatives for Children and Adolescents....................................... Patricia A. Woodbury, C.R.N., M.S.N., C.P.N.A.	59
Chapter 5.	Behavioral Models and Methods for Preventive Health Programs.................................. Robert C. Benfari, Ph.D.	93
Chapter 6.	Practice Management for Clinical Prevention....... G. Frederick Vanderschmidt, Ph.D.	122
Chapter 7.	The Cinderella Effect: Good Teaching Will Transform the Practice of Preventive Medicine..... Hannelore F. Vanderschmidt, Ph.D.	156
Chapter 8.	Health Maintenance in Clinical Practice: An Annotated Review............................. Victoria Logan Lamberton, B.A.	173
Index..		203

CHAPTER I

The Place of the Practice of Clinical Prevention in Health Care

Dieter Koch-Weser, M.D., Ph.D.

The practice of clinical prevention and health maintenance, long neglected and misunderstood, has suddenly entered the mainstream of discussions and even activities in the health field. Despite the spectacular advances in curative medicine, which have increased our life span and decreased suffering and disability, confidence of consumers in the providers of mostly specialized curative care has dwindled to such a degree that much too often the relationship of trust between doctor and patient has been lost. Increased litigation is just one sign of that deplorable development.

Return to primary care and family medicine, which both include a varying degree of attention to preventive care, has been seen by many as a way to reestablish trust between the consumer and the provider of health care.

The World Health Organization definition of health as "physical, mental, and social well-being" and not just the "absence of disease" together with the perhaps utopian goal of "health for all by the year 2000" has contributed to the understanding that maintenance of healthy living conditions that will avoid the onset of disease is at least as important as the cure of disease once it has established itself.

The rapidly escalating cost of curative care, putting it out of reach of many individuals and making it increasingly unaffordable to society as a whole, also has spurred the interest in the practice of clinical prevention.

Those responsible for the organization, administration, and often funding of our health care—federal, state, and local health authorities; as well as insurance companies, health maintenance organizations, labor unions, and health care plans of large corporations have increasingly turned their attention to the potential benefits of establishing health maintenance programs, dedicated to the practice of clinical prevention.

In theory the concept that preventive medicine should be an essential and integral component of clinical practice has been widely accepted. Preventive medicine, however, is not and should not be a separate "specialty." The knowledge, skills, and attitudes which are deemed indispensable to the inclusion of health maintenance and clinical prevention should be part of the arsenal of all health care providers and should be extensively taught, therefore, in all educational and training programs of the health professions.

It must be recognized that together with the health sciences the social sciences play a decisive role in this field, both in education and practice. If present and future health care providers are going to be successful in convincing their patients to participate actively in the prevention of diseases, to adopt a healthier lifestyle, and to be active in health maintenance practices, they must acquire the skills of "social marketing." They must learn how to motivate the public towards better health-related behavior and compliance with measures and activities designed to maintain health. Social, educational, and communication skills, not traditionally a part of health education and practice, must become familar to them.

So far the only curative specialists who have effectively made health maintenance a significant part of their practice are the pediatricians and, to some degree, obstetrician/gynecologists. Among their activities, periodic checkups and prenatal care blend well with the total care of mothers and children. Periodic general examinations of other adults, such as the "yearly executive checkups" quite popular several years ago, have become rare.

It must also be stressed that these checkups, aiming at the early diagnosis of disease processes, mostly in the presymptomatic stages, essentially belong in the category of "secondary prevention." As such, they are intended to treat an already existing pathological condition as early as possible, thereby preventing serious clinical symptoms and disability, as well as irreversible damage. Therefore, in essence, secondary prevention belongs in a good practice of curative medicine. In contrast, "primary prevention" intends to protect the body against even the initial attack and entrance of the disease agent or process.

Infectious diseases provide a good model for differentiation of primary and secondary prevention. Immunization is a primary prevention weapon, blocking the establishment and propagation of an infectious agent within the body. Early diagnosis, for instance by a serological test, and treatment before clincal symptoms appear would constitute secondary prevention.

In some ways, curative and preventive measures are closely related. Early diagnosis and vigorous treatment of an infectious disease, like tuberculosis, are often the most effective primary prevention measures from the public health point of view because they interrupt the chain of transmission and propagation of the disease.

All this brings us to the conclusion that the practice of clinical prevention cannot and should not be isolated from the other forms and modalities of clinical practice. In particular it should be an integral component of primary care and of family practice. It should be blended with and have the same importance as curative activities.

Ample evidence suggests that the trend is in this direction. Not only is it advocated by the health care authorities, but also present and especially future providers recognize that the reliance on curative activities cannot cope with the increasing economic, demographic, and human problems our health care system is facing.

We must also be aware of obstacles and powerful forces opposing change. In addition to the natural inertia in a system and in institutions which leads to resistance to fundamental changes in procedures and values, those who want to dedicate themselves to the practice of clinical prevention will encounter considerable difficulty. They will find that the prestige which the curative specialist enjoys does not necessarily extend to preventive activities. The dramatic cure of a few people from disability and suffering naturally is more impressive than the prevention of a potential, but not yet visible disease by immunization.

Economic rewards for and funding of preventive activities, both at the individual and community levels, are still very scarce. If we lived in a period of expanding support for health care, it probably would be possible to add the cost of clinical prevention to curative health care expenditures. Since that is not the case, some existing curative programs might have to be curtailed to free funds for the addition of preventive care. Such a decision is difficult. Decision makers in our health care system and our teaching institutions learned, practiced, and administered during a period in which biomedical sciences and curative care made unprecedented and highly admirable advances. To deny the enormous benefits which this period brought to our lives and our health would be wrong. We should strive to maintain them and add those aspects of preventive health care which promise to improve the quality of life for all of us in the years to come. The practice of clinical prevention should by no means diminish or substitute for curative health care. Prevention should take its place beside curative care and supplement it.

To that end health professional schools, particularly medical and nursing schools, should emphasize the teaching of clinical prevention. When possible it should occur in settings in which both preventive and curative activities take place. Primary care and family medicine clinics, community health centers, HMOs and other health care facilities in which complete health care for individuals and families is provided, are optimal training sites. Health care providers from different disciplines, such as physicians and nurses, should be trained together because the effective delivery of clinical preventive services depends on teamwork and cooperation.

This book presents the basic components of clinical prevention and how best to organize them for the purpose of developing an effective practice. It is intended for those professionals who wish to devote a significant portion of their time to the practice of clinical prevention.

4   HANDBOOK OF CLINICAL PREVENTION

William H. Barker Jr. indicates why and how epidemiology forms the scientific basis for the practice of clinical prevention and for the achievement of health maintenance.

Joseph Stokes III describes the methods by which health maintenance and health and risk assessment can be achieved and provides advice on how to organize the practice of clinical prevention, its setting, and objectives.

Patricia A. Woodbury emphasizes the importance of clinical preventive initiatives in the development of children and adolescents and how these initiatives fit into primary care activities.

Robert C. Benfari not only descibes the various models and methods of behavioral intervention applied to clinical prevention but also provides detailed examples of intervention sessions.

G. Frederick Vanderschmidt analyzes in some detail the often-neglected management of clinical activities aiming at health maintenance, including staffing, community resource development, and development of income from the practice of clinical prevention.

Hannelore Vanderschmidt outlines the teaching methodology, describing curriculum and course development which differs from the classical classroom and lecture-based teaching model.

Victoria Logan Lamberton reviews the contents of "Health Maintenance in Clinical Practice," an innovative, competency-based instructional series for students and health professionals who wish to explore the topics addressed here in greater depth.

Together with the references given in the various chapters, the editors hope that this book will be a useful tool for those who want to learn about the practice of clinical prevention and those who teach the associated skills and knowledge.

CHAPTER 2

The Epidemiologic Basis of Clinical Prevention

William H. Barker, Jr., M.D.

INTRODUCTION

In its widely accepted role as the fundamental discipline of public health, epidemiology provides the scientific basis for the practice of clinical prevention. Originally defined as "the study of epidemics" (Webster's Dictionary) and largely limited to acute infectious diseases, epidemiology has evolved with the transition to the era of chronic disease and health promotion to encompass the study of distribution, determinants, and deterrents of health and disease.

Distribution refers to the profile of health and disease in a given population, according to the major parameters: time, place, and person. Such information, the byproduct of descriptive epidemiology, is usually expressed in terms of incidence, prevalence, and mortality rates.

Determinants constitute those etiologic agents, risk factors, or predisposing conditions of health and disease which are elucidated by analytic epidemiology. Analytic studies yield information on the validity and strength of association between risk factors and the occurrence of a disease.

Deterrents consist of individual and community interventions to maintain or improve health by modifying or reducing exposure to established etiologic agents and risk factors. Epidemiology contributes to knowledge regarding effectiveness and efficiency of such deterrents by guiding the design and conduct of intervention studies—both experimental and quasi-experimental—in populations.

The purpose of this chapter is to review ways in which these precepts of epidemiology, employed in studying events in populations, provide clinicians with essential information and tools for practicing health maintenance in individuals.

EXPANDING THE MEDICAL MODEL

The classic biomedical model which has dominated the teaching and practice of clinical medicine in the twentieth century consists of (see Figure 2.1):

- an encounter between a patient with signs and symptoms and a physician armed with biomedical knowledge and technology;
- diagnosis of a specific disease or condition;
- treatment with medicine or surgery; and
- cure as the expected result.

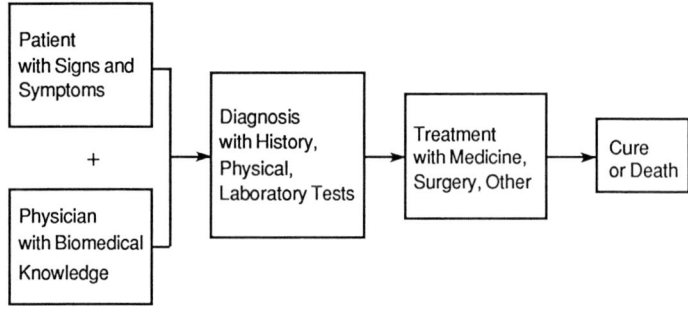

Figure 2.1. Traditional biomedical model of clinical practice.

While this reactive and reductionist model is quite ample for defining the curative component of medical practice, it is insufficient for accommodating the largely anticipatory functions required in practicing health promotion and disease prevention, i.e. clinical health maintenance. The latter requires a model of medical practice such as depicted in Figure 2.2, which envisions the provider defining the practice population; considering the health risks most likely to threaten members of that population within various age and sex strata; becoming familiar and familiarizing associates with the current state of knowledge with regard to preventing or deterring ill consequences of such health risks; and planning and implementing strategies within the practice setting to assure optimal provision of the fruits of this knowledge, tailored to the needs of individual members of the practice population. The actual delivery or provision of health maintenance services to the individual as envisioned in this model requires a variety of managerial and communication skills which are discussed in subsequent chapters of this book. Underlying the entire process is a rich and essential set of contributions from epidemiology.[1]

The following sections delineate this epidemiologic base of clinical prevention, first from the perspective of the broad determinants of health status and then from the perspective of two major subdivisions of disease: the acute infectious diseases, largely caused by single, specific microbial agents; and the chronic diseases, usually caused by multiple and often nonspecific or unknown factors. A final section briefly discusses practical methods for incorporating current epidemiologic knowledge from these several broad areas into practice-based clinical prevention programs.

DETERMINANTS OF HEALTH STATUS

Health has been defined by the Association of Teachers of Preventive Medicine as a state characterized by anatomic integrity; ability to perform personal valued roles; ability to deal with physical, biological and social stress; and freedom from presence or risk of disease and untimely death. Health status in a given individual may be measured in terms of a number of qualities, including immunization history, presence of or exposure to known health risks, reserve capacity of specific organ systems to respond to demand, evidence of preclinical or clinical disease, ability to perform essential activities of daily living (feeding, dressing, ambulation, etc.), and affective and cognitive mental function.[2]

Historical and contemporary epidemiologic observations have lead to the recognition that a person's health status is determined by influences from four broad domains:

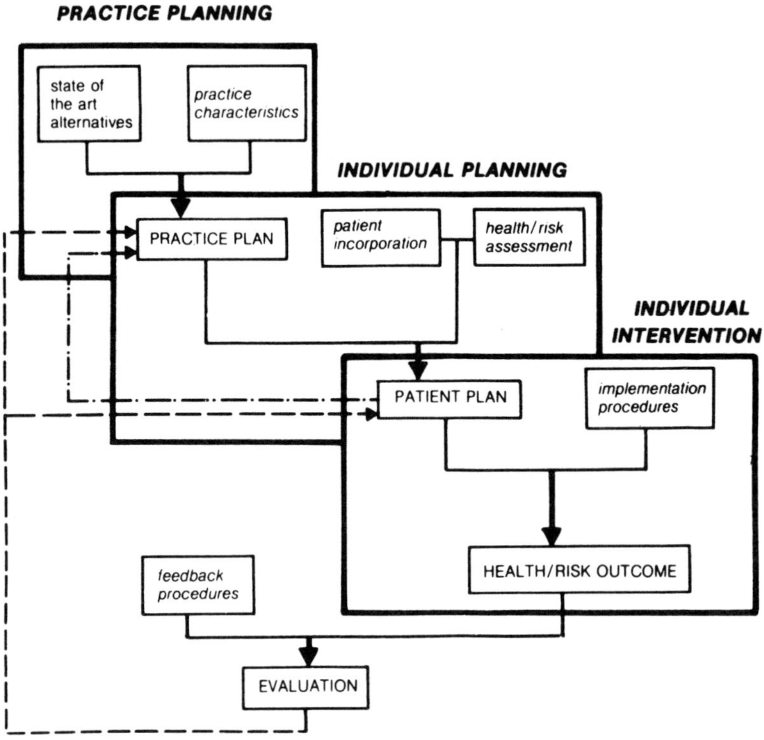

From: Segall A, Barker WH, Cobb S, Jackson G, Noren J, Shindell S, Stokes J III, Ericsson S: Development of a competency-based approach to teaching preventive medicine. Preventive Medicine, 1981;10:726-735. Reprinted by permission.

Figure 2.2. A model for planning and implementing clinical health maintenance in a medical practice.

- Heredity: the genetic traits with which an individual is endowed at birth;
- Environment: one's physical, sociocultural, and occupational milieu;
- Lifestyle: personal habits or behaviors that one either does or does not adopt;
- Medical Care: preventive, curative, rehabilitative, and supportive services.

In considering the clinician's role with respect to health maintenance in the individual, it is well to recognize opportunities to positively affect an individual's health through efforts directed at one or more of these four broad areas of health determinants. In addition it is well to recognize and, where possible, contribute in a positive way to other broad societal forces which are conducive to good health. Two provocative theses in this regard are contained in the recent writings of McKeown[3] and Fries.[4] The former attributes most of the decline in mortality and improvement in health in the past to nonmedical, largely social and economic events, while the latter optimistically forecasts a future in which people will live a relatively disease—and disability—free life ("rectangularizing of morbidity") as a consequence of adopting more healthful lifestyles.

ACUTE INFECTIOUS DISEASE

While infectious respiratory tract and gastro-intestinal diseases once topped the list of causes of death in our society, such mortality has been dramatically reduced through the fruits of environmental hygiene, improved nutrition, specific immunizing agents and antibiotics (see Table 2.1). Nonetheless infections remain common causes of preventable morbidity and in the case of pneumonia and influenza, a continuing leading cause of preventable mortality among elderly persons with chronic disease.

Table 2.1
Leading Causes of Death in the United States 1900 and 1980

1900	1980
Influenza and pneumonia	Heart disease
Tuberculosis	Malignant neoplasms
Diarrhea and related diseases	Stroke
Heart disease	Accidents, poisoning
Stroke	Influenza and pneumonia

10 HANDBOOK OF CLINICAL PREVENTION

An epidemiological model for understanding the dynamics and potentials for protecting individuals and communities against acute communicable diseases is depicted in Figure 2.3. The essential elements in this model comprise a pathogenic <u>agent</u>, a susceptible <u>host</u>, and an <u>environment</u> which facilitates transmission of the agent to the host.

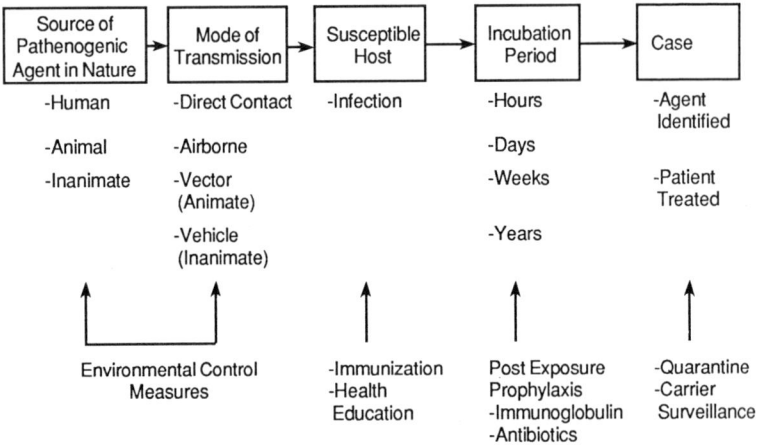

Figure 2.3. Dynamics of communicable disease epidemiology and prevention.

In brief the presence of a pathogenic agent in the animate or inanimate environment (eg, Salmonella in meat and poultry) and the exposure of a susceptible individual (eg, anyone, particularly the very young and very old) to an infecting dose of the agent by way of one of several modes of transmission (eg, cross-contamination or inadequate cooking of food) leads to infection. Following an incubation period, which may vary from hours to weeks, depending upon the speed with which the agent's pathogenic effects occur, (eg, two-three days for most Salmonella gastroenteritis), the disease becomes clinically manifest in the host.

Successful measures to prevent or control spread of specific communicable diseases are dependent upon a knowledge of the various agent, host, and environmental dynamics peculiar to each such disease. From the point of view of the clinical practitioner, it would be most important to know which persons (by age, sex, occupation, etc.) in one's practice and practice setting, are most susceptible to incurring which communicable diseases. In turn one should be well acquainted with appropriate preventive measures to offer to those at risk for a given disease. These would most frequently consist of providing immunizations as part of routine practice, in accord with current recommendations for a given age group. Also important with respect to certain communicable diseases would be the provision of postexposure prophylactic therapy with immunoglobulin, antibiotics, and antivirals to persons at risk of secondary spread of the disease. Examples include gamma globulin for household contacts of infectious (type A) hepatitis, rifampin for household and day care contacts of patients with meningococcal or Hemophilus influenzae infections, and amantadine for high risk individuals (e.g. nursing home residents) exposed to influenza A.

While clinical practitioners are less likely to become directly involved with the environmental aspects of communicable disease control, they nonetheless play an important role in reporting unusual cases or clusters of cases to local health authorities. This in turn may lead to epidemiologic investigation and implementation of environmental control measures where indicated. Significant outbreaks of foodbourne disease, hepatitis, zoonotic disease, and other acute public health problems with possible environmental cause are often first recognized through such reporting. The following standard sources contain essential epidemiology and recommended preventive procedures for virtually all communicable diseases likely to be encountered in the United States and in travel abroad:

- Control of Communicable Disease in Man—a clearly organized practical manual compiled and updated every three to five years by a committee of experts and published by the American Public Health Association, Washington, DC;
- Report of the Committee on Infectious Diseases—American Academy of Pediatrics, Evanston, IL. Updated periodically;
- Guide for Adult Immunization—prepared by the Committee on Immunization, American College of Physicians, Philadelphia, PA;
- Health Information for International Travelers—Guidelines issued periodically and available on request from the Centers for Disease Control, Atlanta, GA 30333;
- The Morbidity and Mortality Weekly Report (MMWR)—published by the U.S. Public Health Service, Centers for Disease Control. This publication contains timely information on current patterns of communicable disease nationally and regionally, plus periodic revisions of recommendations for vaccination (eg, annual influenza vaccination guidelines), and other approaches to control of diseases of public health concern. The MMWR has played an essential role in the present decade in disseminating information on acquired immune deficiency syndrome (AIDS), including definition of high risk groups, recommendations regarding candidates for screening, and approaches to prevention.

(Note: Many state, county and city health departments publish similar periodic disease control bulletins focusing on the epidemiologic status of communicable disease at a more local level.)

CHRONIC DISEASE—NATURAL HISTORY

The major "killers and cripplers" of contemporary society are the chronic diseases. In contrast to most communicable diseases, chronic diseases are generally the result of a protracted period of pathogenesis, occurring over years rather than the hours, days, or weeks of incubation in communicable diseases. Etiology is generally multifactorial with poorly understood interactions among factors; is best characterized as a "web of causality" in contrast to the somewhat simpler "chain of causality" involved in the transmission of a specific infectious agent in communicable diseases. New cases tend to occur relatively infrequently in a steady endemic pattern in contrast to the tendency for acute communicable diseases to occur in clusters, occasionally in epidemic form, and often with some seasonal pattern.

The "natural history of disease" model shown in Figure 2.4 serves as a useful paradigm for summarizing knowledge about the evolution of a given chronic disease in the individual and for considering possible opportunities for preventive interventions. The upper part of the model portrays a series of indentifiable stages of disease development and the traditional measurable manifestations of each stage. The lower part depicts the potential interventions—specific tactics and broad practice strategies—which might be used to prevent or deter progression at each stage.

Of primary interest in the practice of prevention are the first two stages, those of "nondisease" and "biologic onset," during which individuals while ostensibly healthy, are in fact exposed to "risks" or possessed of harbingers ("signs") of clinically manifest disease which may be in the offing.

Primary preventive interventions, directed at reducing or avoiding exposure to risk factors, may take a variety of forms, including health education, behavior modification, and legislated social policy. Examples include nutritional counseling and smoking cessation programs to help individuals reduce their risk of developing coronary artery disease and state laws that require seat belt use or raise the legal drinking age in order to prevent highway deaths and crippling injuries.

Secondary prevention is premised upon the ability through laboratory screening to detect significant physiological or morphological abnormalities and to intervene medically or surgically to eliminate or control the abnormality prior to the development of symptomatic disease. Amniocentesis for detecting genetic disease, Papanicolaou testing for cervical carcinoma, and blood pressure monitoring to detect hypertension —each followed by the appropriate therapeutic response to positive findings—exemplify the range of applications of secondary prevention.

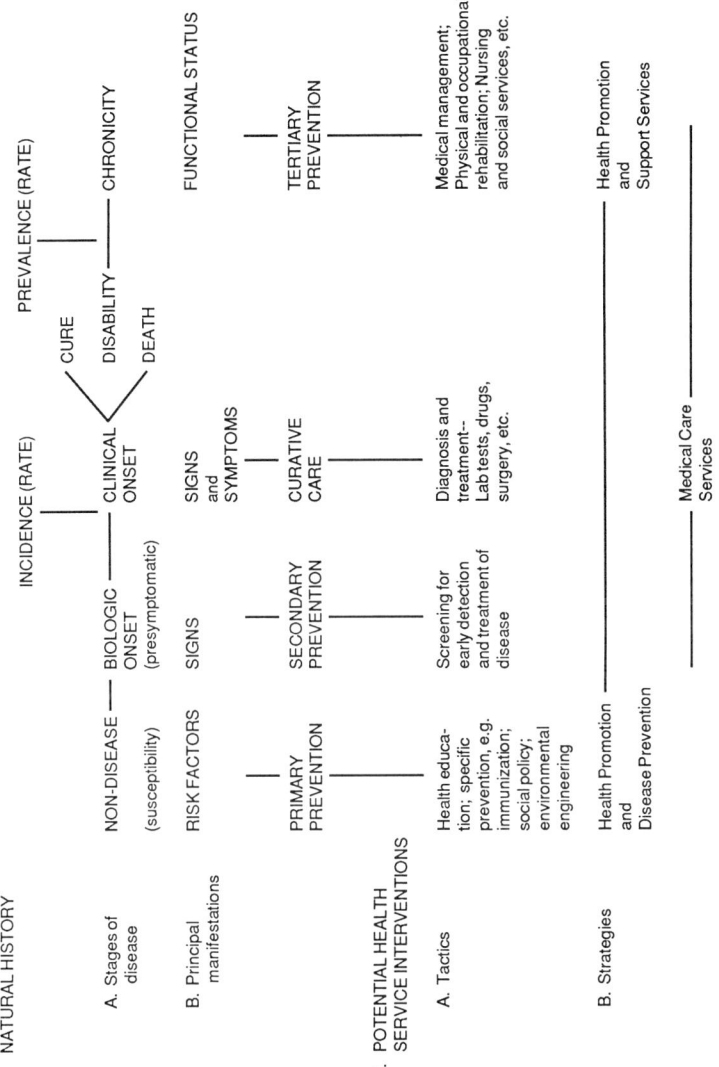

Figure 2.4. The natural history of disease and potential health service interventions.

RISK FACTORS AND PRIMARY PREVENTION

The concept of risk factors in chronic disease emerged from the Framingham Study which was undertaken by the U.S. Public Health Service in the 1950s to elucidate associations between various personal and environmental attributes and the occurrence of cardiovascular diseases. As pointed out in a recent review article by William Kannel[5], director of the Framingham Study for a number of years, "risk factors" as defined in epidemiological studies represent statistical associations between the presence of a given factor and the occurrence of a disease; hence, they may be directly causative, secondary manifestations of more basic underlying metabolic abnormalities, or early symptoms of the disease.

Significance of a given risk factor in causing or predisposing to a disease may be expressed in terms of absolute risk, relative risk, or attributable risk. A high relative risk, comparing incidence of disease among those with and without the factor of interest may mean little from the practice population perspective if the absolute risk (ie, annual incidence of disease) is low or the occurrence of the risk factor in the population at large is so infrequent that the amount of disease that is attributable to the factor (ie, population attributable risk) is low.

Through a hierarchy of epidemiologic and related studies, hypotheses regarding exposure to risk factors for specific disease are generated and tested (Table 2.2). Descriptive epidemiologic studies define incidence rates (occurrence of new cases over time in a defined population) and prevalence rates (extant cases in a population at a given point or period of time), often suggesting an association between certain personal or environmental attributes and occurrence of disease. Analytic epidemiologic studies, drawing upon suggested associations from clinical and pathological observations as well as descriptive epidemiology, are designed to compare the incidence of disease among groups with and without a hypothesized risk factor. These studies are generally conducted using either a cohort or case control study design.

Table 2.2
Hierarchy of Epidemiological and Related Clinical Studies Used to Elucidate Disease Causality

INDIVIDUALS	POPULATIONS
Clinical case reports	Descriptive statistics
Pathologic observations	Ecological associations
	Cross-sectional surveys
	Case control study
	Cohort study
	Quasi-experimental interventions
	Experimental interventions - randomized clinical trial

In a cohort study, which requires a relatively long period of time (five to ten years), a population of persons, some exposed to the risk factor(s) of interest and some without, or with varying degrees of exposure (eg, varying levels of serum cholesterol) is followed over time to compare the incidence of new cases of disease among groups.

In a case control study, which can be completed in a relatively short period of time (a year or less), with relatively few study subjects, persons with the disease under study (cases) are compared with otherwise similar persons without the disease (controls), to determine whether the former are more likely to have been exposed to the risk factor of interest prior to occurrence of the disease. Table 2.3 lists a number of examples of hypothesized causal or risk relations to major chronic diseases which have been investigated using cohort and case control studies.

Table 2.3
Examples of Cohort and Case-Control Studies to Generate and Test Causal Hypotheses for Major Chronic Diseases

STUDY TYPE	DISEASES, CONDITIONS	HYPOTHESIZED CAUSES RISK FACTORS
Cohort	Coronary artery disease	Hypertension, cholesterol, smoking, etc.
Cohort	Lung cancer	Smoking
Cohort	Multiple cancers	Radiation exposure
Cohort	Low birthweight infants	Smoking, alcohol, status, etc.
Case Control	Vaginal adenocarcinoma	Diethylstilbestrol
Case Control	Uterine cancer	Exogenous estrogen
Case Control	Pancreatic cancer	Coffee
Case Control	Colon cancer	Cholecystectomy
Case Control	Bleeding gastric ulcer	Nonsteroid anti-inflammatory drugs

Note: Some of the hypotheses listed here have been substantiated while others have not.

The ultimate test of a risk factor's role in disease causation emerges from intervention trials wherein a group in which the factor is reduced or eliminated is compared with a similar group in which the factor is not reduced or eliminated. If in fact the occurrence of the target disease is significantly reduced among the former, a causal role for the risk factor may be assumed. The value of a particular intervention in preventing the target disease among persons receiving the intervention is computed as "percent effectiveness," using the following basic formula:

$$(1- \text{Observed Incidence}/\text{Expected Incidence}) \times 100$$

Thus in one of the Veterans Administration studies[6] of controlling high blood pressure, 18% of the treated group experienced cardiovascular complications of hypertension versus 55% among the control group. Effectiveness of this preventive intervention was thereby computed as follows:

$$(1-18/55) \times 100 = 67\%$$

CARDIOVASCULAR DISEASE EPIDEMIOLOGY

The contribution of epidemiologic studies of risk factors to planning a practice-based health maintenance strategy may be illustrated with several findings from cardiovascular disease epidemiology.

Of fundamental importance from the Framingham and other longitudinal studies of the natural history of cardiovascular diseases has been the recognition and quantification of the increased risk associated with multiple, independent risk factors. In turn, the cumulative risk from one or more risk factors, and from increasing levels of each of these, has been quantified. A typical summary statement from such data is depicted in Figure 2.5, compiled from Framingham data, which shows the increasing probability of experiencing cardiovascular disease for an individual at a given age, dependent upon risk factor status. Such data have been incorporated into Stroke and Coronary Risk Handbooks (published by the American Heart Association) and other formats for easy reference in determining the risk status of individual patients in the practice setting.

A number of experimental and quasi-experimental studies undertaken in recent years are in turn yielding useful information regarding effectiveness of clinical preventive interventions in reducing cardiovascular risk factors. These include the Veterans Administration Hypertension Studies,[6] the Multiple Risk Factor Intervention Trial (MRFIT),[7] the Hypertension Detection and Follow-up Program (HDFP),[8] the Stanford Heart Disease Prevention Program,[9] the Lipid Research Clinic Trials(LRC),[10] and the Systolic Hypertension in the Elderly Program (SHEP).[11] While the results of these and related studies in other countries are too numerous to summarize, principles of epidemiological analysis in interpreting and applying results to individuals and communities may be appreciated from several examples.

First is the fundamental need to distinguish between the significance of <u>relative risk</u> and <u>absolute risk</u> in deciding practice priorities for targeting preventive services. This is clearly illustrated in an important article by Geoffrey Rose,[12] a distinguished British epidemiologist, who shows graphically that relative risk for mortality increases with increasing levels of blood pressure among all age groups; however, the gradient of increased relative risk across blood pressure levels lessens as age advances. If one were to target preventive efforts according to relative risk gradients, priorities for hypertension detection and treatment would be directed to younger adults. However, examining

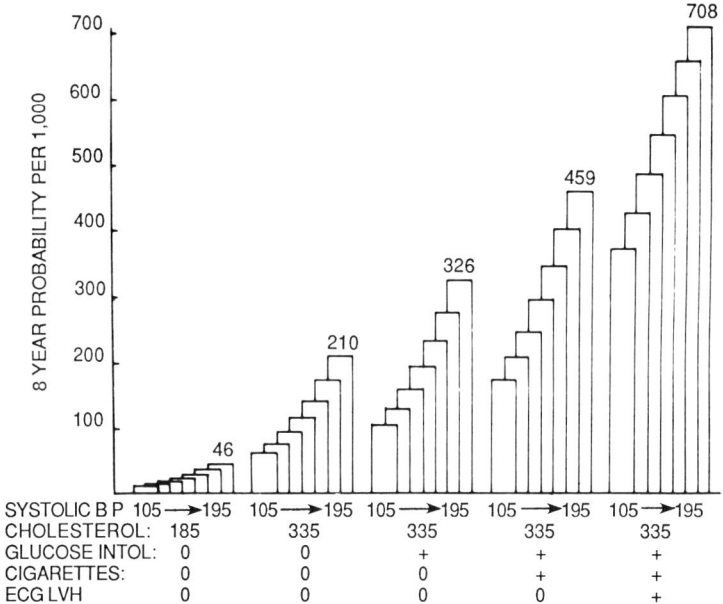

From: Kannel WB: Chapter 1: An overview of the risk factors for cardiovascular disease. IN: Kaplan NM and Stamler J (eds.): Prevention of Coronary Heart Disease. Philadelphia, PA: WB Saunders, 1983. Reprinted by permission.

Figure 2.5. Effect of multiple risk factors on occurrence of cardiovascular disease. The eight year probability per 1000 men aged 40 of cardiovascular disease according to systolic blood pressures from 105 to 195 mm Hg at specified levels of other risk factors. From the Framingham Study monograph No. 28.

absolute risk of mortality reveals that this is far higher for older persons than younger persons at each level of blood pressure. Furthermore, a higher percentage of older persons have blood pressures at the higher end of the range. These data would argue for prioritizing hypertension detection and treatment to older members of one's practice.[12]

The argument for focusing on absolute versus relative risk is in fact borne out in data from the V.A. trials of antihypertensive treatment in which effectiveness of treatment expressed in relative terms was around 50-60% regardless of age or presence of comorbidities, but due to their greater absolute risk, the benefits in terms of cardiovascular events (strokes, etc.) prevented per 100 hypertensive persons treated were more than twice as great for those over age 50 than for those under age 50 (Table 2.4).

Table 2.4
Relative (Column A) and Absolute (Column B) Benefits from the Treatment of Hypertension According to Age and the Presence of Cardiovascular-Renal Abnormality

AGE (YRS)	CARDIOVASCULAR - RENAL ABNORMALITY	A TREATMENT EFFECTIVENESS (%)	B EVENTS PREVENTED PER 100 TREATED
<50	absent	59	6
	present	62	14
>50	absent	50	15
	present	60	29

From: Veterans Administration Cooperative Study Group on Antihypertension Agents: Effects of treatment on morbidity in hypertension. Circulation, 1972;45:991-1004. Reprinted by permission of the American Heart Association, Inc.

A further excellent illustration of the value of epidemiology in determining who is most likely or least likely to benefit from preventive intervention is found in the analysis of mortality results of the MRFIT study. Overall findings with respect to the study's primary end point, coronary heart disease (CHD) mortality, are summarized in Table 2.5.

Table 2.5
MRFIT: Differences in Coronary Heart Disease (CHD) Mortality Between Special Intervention (SI) and Usual Care (UC) Among Study Subgroups

SUBGROUPS	PERCENT DIFFERENCE IN CHD MORTALITY, SI vs. UC
All men	-7.1
All nonhypertensives	-21.1
Hypertensives with normal baseline ECG	-23.7
Hypertensives with abnormal baseline ECG	+65

From: Multiple Risk Factor Intervention Trial Research Group: Multiple risk factor intervention trial. Journal of the American Medical Association, 1982;248:1465-1477. Copyright 1982, American Medical Association. Reprinted by permission.

While a reduction of about 22% was expected among the special multiple risk factor intervention (SI) group in comparison with the usual care control group, the observed reduction in the SI group was only 7.1%. On further analysis by subgroup, it was found that among those SI subjects who were either nonhypertensive or were hypertensive but had normal electrocardiograms (ECG) (who between them represented 81% of the group) CHD mortality was in fact reduced by 21-23%. However, among the 19% of SI subjects with hypertension and abnormal ECGs, there was an unexpected 65% increase in CHD mortality. The force of this negative outcome was sufficient to yield the resultant disappointingly low 7.1% effectiveness for the SI group as a whole. These findings on the one hand support the value of an organized multiple risk factor detection and reduction program, including antihypertensive treatment for those hypertensives with normal ECGs; on the other hand they alert practitioners to the likely risk of using antihypertensives (particularly diuretic agents) in treating that substantial subgroup of hypertensive patients with abnormal ECGs.[7]

In addition to its role in assessing effectiveness of specific preventive intervention tactics, as illustrated above, epidemiology plays an important role in evaluating the effectiveness of practice strategies in successfully implementing preventive interventions. The results of a study of the effectiveness of a community oriented primary care (COPC) practice, as compared to usual primary care (PC), in controlling high blood pressure are summarized in Table 2.6, adapted from the work of Sidney Kark and colleagues.[14] COPC, the practice strategy under study, consists of a primary care practice in which the population is well defined; curative, preventive, and health promotion services are integrated; health care needs of the population and the success with which they are being met are continuously monitored; and practice operations are modified to address unmet needs. As noted in Table 2.6, prevalence rates of uncontrolled hypertension decreased to considerably greater degrees in COPC subjects in most age-sex groups over the five year period of the study. Such data would argue in favor of adopting elements of the COPC strategy in one's own practice as a means to attaining successful preventive outcomes. (The model shown in Figure 2.2 may be thought of as depicting the preventive component of a COPC strategy.)

SCREENING AND SECONDARY PREVENTION

The concept of early diagnosis and intervention in disease process (secondary prevention) has been advocated for several decades. Successes with detection and therapeutic intervention in the presymptomatic, early biologic stage of tuberculosis (chest x-rays) and cervical carcinoma (Pap smear test) in the 1950s have been followed by the development of screening tests for many other chronic conditions. These have been in turn incorporated into a variety of health maintenance packages tailored according to age and sex. Since screening tests are intended for use in large numbers of healthy people, they tend to be relatively simple and inexpensive. Accordingly, they are generally less accurate or definitive than traditional full medical evaluation in making diagnoses.

Table 2.6
Change in Prevalence Rates of Uncontrolled Hypertension per 100 Persons by Age and Sex in COPC and the Control Populations

	COPC				CONTROL-PC ONLY			
	MEN		WOMEN		MEN		WOMEN	
Age	Initial Survey	5-Year Survey	Initial Survey	5-Year Survey	Initial Survey	5-Year Survey	Initial Survey	5-Year Survey
35-44	11.3	6.5	13.6	6.2	9.6	6.4	8.9	7.3
45-54	22.9	8.9	23.9	15.9	20.7	14.6	17.9	12.5
55-64	35.1	24.6	36.8	27.6	28.2	23.0	32.9	33.5
65-74	36.4	27.3	43.2	43.2	36.7	33.3	48.1	40.7

From: Abramson JH and Kark SL: Community-oriented primary care: Meaning and scope. IN: Connor E and Mullen F: Community Oriented Primary Care. Washington, DC: National Academy Press, 1983. Reprinted by permission.

Epidemiology contributes to the development and interpretation of secondary prevention in several ways of importance to planning a clinical health maintenance program. These include defining screening tests in terms of their accuracy (sensitivity and specificity) and efficiency (predictive value) in detecting disease, evaluating the impact of a given screening test or screening package on the health of a population of screenees in terms of reduction in morbidity and mortality, and defining which subgroups of the population are most likely to benefit from specific screening tests.

CHARACTERIZING A SCREENING TEST

The sensitivity and specificity of a screening test in yielding an accurate final diagnosis are best appreciated in Table 2.7 which distributes subjects according to their true final diagnosis (often referred to as the "gold standard") and their diagnosis according to the screening test under study. The letter $\underline{a}$ denotes persons with the disease who were correctly classified by the screening test while $\underline{b}$ represents persons without disease who were diagnosed to have disease (false positives). The letter $\underline{c}$ denotes truly diseased persons whom the screening test failed to detect (false negatives) while $\underline{d}$ represents those without disease who were correctly classified by the screening test.

Sensitivity and specificity are computed as shown by the formulas:

$$\text{Sensitivity} = a / a + c$$

and

$$\text{Specificity} = d / b + d.$$

Table 2.7
Relationship of Screening-Test Results to True Diagnosis

SCREENING TEST	TRUE DIAGNOSIS		TOTAL
	DISEASE PRESENT	DISEASE ABSENT	
Positive	a	b	a + b
Negative	c	d	c + d
Total	a + c	b + d	a + b + c + d

Sensitivity = a / a + c
Specificity = d / b + d

a = persons with disease and correctly diagnosed
b = persons without disease but diagnosed as having disease (false positives)
c = persons with disease but diagnosed as not having disease (false negatives)
d = persons without disease and correctly diagnosed

Both of these are of concern in practicing preventive care. Sensitivity indicates how completely one can expect to detect, hence intervene, early on all true cases, while specificity measures the degree to which one is correctly classifying well persons and avoiding the unnecessary anxiety and costly followup evaluation of false positives.

Predictive value positive (PVP), the proportion of positive screenees that are true positives (a / a + b), provides an estimate of the efficiency of a screening test. It is important to appreciate that if a disease is relatively infrequent in the population, as is the case with most chronic diseases, even a screening test with a high degree of specificity will yield a sizeable number of false positives. This in turn will lower the predictive value of a positive test. Possible approaches to alter the use of a screening test toward a higher PVP are discussed in a public health monograph by Thorner and Remein.[15]

Table 2.8, shows the results of screening for diabetes mellitus in a hypothetical population of 10,000 persons with a true diabetes prevalence rate of 1.5%. Screening for blood glucose with a cutoff point of 130 mg/100 ml, which had a sensitivity of 44.3% and a specificity of 99.0%, yielded the results shown in part A. Notably, of the 164 screen positives, 98 were in fact false positives; PVP was therefore 40% (66/164). Predictive value would be significantly improved by defining the screening cutoff point at a higher level, 180 mg/ ml at which level specificity increases to 99.8%. Of the 54 screen positives, 34 are correct, giving a more efficient PVP of 63%. However, there is a marked drop in sensitivity as only 34 of 150 (22.3%) true diabetics are detected.

Table 2.8
Results of Screening for Diabetes Mellitus on a Hypothetical Population of 10,000 Using Two Different Cutoff Points

A. Cutoff Point = 130 mg%

SCREENING TEST	TRUE DIAGNOSIS		TOTAL
	DIABETIC	NOT DIABETIC	
Positive	66	98	164
Negative	84	9,752	9,836
Total	150	9,850	10,000

(Disease prevalence = 1.5%, Sensitivity = 44.3%, Specificity = 99.0%)

B. Cutoff Point = 180 mg%

SCREENING TEST	TRUE DIAGNOSIS		TOTAL
	DIABETIC	NOT DIABETIC	
Positive	34	20	54
Negative	116	9,830	9,946
Total	150	9,850	10,000

(Disease prevalence = 1.5%, Sensitivity = 22.3%, Specificity = 99.8%)

From: Thorner RM and Remein QR: Principles and Procedures in the Evaluation of Screening for Disease. U.S. Public Health Monograph, 1961; No. 67.

Predictive value may also be improved, without necessarily sacrificing sensitivity, by directing screening tests to a subgroup of the population with known higher disease prevalence, under which circumstances a larger proportion of screen positives will be true positives. This might be achieved in the case of diabetes by targeting high risk persons such as those who are obese or who have family history of the disease.

EVALUATING HEALTH IMPACT OF SCREENING

The ultimate value of a screening test, once incorporated into practice at a given level of sensitivity, specificity, and predictive value is its demonstrated ability to reduce mortality or morbidity when compared with usual medical care, without screening intervention. This question of preventive effectiveness is best answered through formal clinical trials, designed in ways analagous to those discussed above for risk factor reduction programs. Brief summary of two such trials, one dealing with screening for a single disease (breast cancer), the other dealing with a periodic multi-phasic screening program, are illustrative.

In the mid-1960s, a randomized clinical trial of the benefits of annual screening for breast cancer with mammography and clinical examination was undertaken involving 62,000 women who were enrolled in the Health Insurance Plan of Greater New York. Comparison over a number of years of the 31,000 women who received the program with the 31,000 controls revealed a higher rate of newly diagnosed cases of breast cancer and higher percentages of cancers without evidence of spread to axillary lymph nodes. While these early findings were encouraging, the proof of the pudding was whether or not mortality was reduced among the screenees. That this was the case is shown in a summary of mortality data shown in Table 2.9. Importantly, however, on subgroup analysis it is apparent that benefits of this breast cancer screening program (annual mammography and clinical examination) were only found in women over age 50.[16]

Table 2.9
Breast Cancer Mortality Among Study and Control Groups by Age, Five Year Followup, H.I.P. Screening Program

	DEATHS PER 10,000	
AGE GROUP	STUDY	CONTROL
40-49	2.5	2.4
50-59	2.3	5.0
60-69	3.4	5.0

From: Shapiro S: Evidence for screening for breast cancer from a randomized trial. Cancer, supplement 1977;39:2772-2782. Reprinted by permission.

Also in the 1960s, a controlled trial was undertaken by the Kaiser-Permanente Medical Care Plan in northern California to assess the overall benefit of the popular but controversial practice of periodic multiphasic medical screening. A systematic sampling of the Plan's membership yielded two similar groups of over 5,000 men and women between 35 and 54 years of age. The study group was encouraged to receive annual multiphasic testing, including screening tests for a number of conditions, while the control group received usual medical care (including screening if requested). Results over the first decade indicated that significantly more disease had been diagnosed and treated in the study group. Evidence of reduced disability and reduced mortality from certain detectable diseases (hypertension-related deaths, colon cancer) was initially apparent only in the subgroup of men aged 45 to 54 at the outset of the study. Studies in other settings have not demonstrated significantly better health outcomes among persons receiving multiphasic screening compared with control groups.[17]

Thus, while the value of a full screening program or annual checkup has not been convincingly proven, a number of specific screening procedures are certainly of demonstrated value when targeted to the right subgroup of the population. A breast cancer screening program targeted to women over age 50 would be a case in point, as would be a screening program for blood lead levels targeted to young children living in old houses known to harbor lead paint.

PRACTICE HEALTH MAINTENANCE STRATEGIES

Three epidemiologically based tasks are required in adopting a health maintenance plan in clinical practice as envisioned in the model described at the beginning of this chapter.

State of the Art Alternatives

The first task is to review the current state of knowledge regarding health risks or early signs of disease which may be prevented or modified through either primary or secondary prevention in the clinical setting. Rather than undertaking a major literature review and assessment on one's own, it is advisable to consult one of a number of reliable syntheses of the state of the art which are currently available. Examples of such available sources include:

a. Report of Canadian Task Force on Periodic Health Examination[18]
   This document is periodically updated by a committee of experts and widely disseminated in the United States as well as Canada. It contains the results of a careful assessment of epidemiologic and related evidence with regard to effectiveness and appropriateness of a large series of potentially useful primary and secondary preventive practices for persons according to age.

b. An analogous review prepared and recently updated by Dr. Paul Frame,[19] a family practitioner with a long-standing interest and widely recognized expertise in incorporating health maintenance into primary care practice.

c. Guidelines for Cancer-Related Checkup,[20] prepared and periodically updated by the American Cancer Society. Screening recommendations by age and sex are provided on a summary chart, accompanied by a useful review of the evidence and rationale for each test.

Practice Population Characteristics

This task is intended to provide an estimate of the number (or proportion) of one's patients likely to be candidates for various health maintenance services which one might wish to provide on the basis of the aforementioned review of the state of the art. Since age and sex are the two most readily accessible population characteristics that relate to the distribution of risk factors and disease, it is helpful to have an age-sex register of one's patient population. If this is not available, an estimate might be made. With this practice demographic profile in hand it is possible to estimate the number of persons for whom a given preventive intervention might be indicated. For example, for various cardiovascular disease risk factors one might apply age-specific prevalence rates to respective age-sex groups in one's practice population such as shown in Table 2.10. Such simple quantification will provide guidance for prioritizing health maintenance services.

Table 2.10
Estimated Number of Persons with Selected Cardiovascular Risk Factors in a Family Practice Population, Utilizing National Age-Sex Prevalence Rates (Shown in Parentheses)

	AGE				
	15-24	25-44	45-64	>64	TOTAL
Total Population	2918	5969	1552	784	11223
Males	1181	2614	679	271	4745
Females	1737	3355	873	513	6478
Smokers [†]					
Males	461 (39%)	1124 (43%)	278 (41%)	49 (18%)	1912
Females	573 (33%)	1107 (33%)	271 (31%)	87 (17%)	2038
Hypertensive [††]					
Males	35 (3%)	288 (11%)	197 (29%)	103 (38%)	623
Females	17 (1%)	235 (7%)	271 (31%)	267 (52%)	790
Hypercholesteremia [†††]					
Males		471 (18%)	149 (22%)	49 (18%)	669
Females		503 (15%)	253 (29%)	180 (35%)	936

[†] Prevalence rates derived from National Health Interview Survey, 1980.
[††] Prevalence rates derived from Health and Nutritional Evaluation Survey, 1976 - 1980.
[†††] Prevalence rates derived from N.I.H. Consensus Development Conference on Lowering Blood Cholesterol, 1984.

From: Unpublished data prepared by Kathleen Jewel, MD using Population Register of University of Rochester Family Medicine Center. Used by permission.

Prevalence rates from national survey data obtained with assistance of Carol Haines, MPH, Health Education Branch, National Heart, Lung and Blood Institute.

Aids to Implementation

A variety of useful aids might be employed to facilitate implementation of epidemiologically indicated preventive practices. These range from various disease-specific tactics to health hazard appraisal instruments directed at a broad range of preventable problems. Examples include:

- Influenza—postcards sent to patients in high risk groups (eg, elderly with chronic cardiac, pulmonary, renal and other conditions) have been shown in a number of settings to markedly enhance the percent receiving recommended annual vaccination.[21]
- Coronary Artery Disease and Stroke—American Heart Association risk handbooks allow one to readily determine for an individual of a given age and sex the summation of risk conferred by all of the major cardiovascular risk factors.[22]
- Health Hazard or Risk Appraisal—Self-administered comprehensive questionnaire which assembles an individual's major health risk data. Computerized analysis provides statements regarding one's risks of premature death and an estimate of benefits (in terms of longevity) to be realized from modifying specific risks. The Centers for Disease Control have developed such an instrument for general use and a number of commercial versions are also becoming available.

Formal surveys and anecdotal information from many sources attest to a high level of current interest on the part of both medical professionals and the public at large in seeing disease prevention and health promotion incorporated more vigorously into medical practice. A working acquaintance with principles of epidemiology and their application in clinical practice, reviewed in this chapter, is an essential first step toward accomplishing that end. Experiences in which these have been successfully applied constitute important models for others to learn from. Several such exemplary models, ranging from a rural office-based family medicine practice to an urban health maintenance organization have been described and are commended to the aspiring practitioner of clinical prevention.[23]

REFERENCES

1. Segall AJ, Jackson GW, Barker WH, et al: Physician performance objectives: A basis for preventive medicine curriculum development. IN: Barker W (ed.): Teaching Preventive Medicine in Primary Care. New York: Springer Publishing Co., 1983, Chapter 6.

2. Stokes J, Noren J and Shindell S: Definition of terms and concepts applicable to clinical preventive medicine. J Community Health 1982;8:33-41.

3. McKeown T: The Role of Medicine: Dream, Mirage or Nemesis? London: Nuffield Hospitals Trust, 1976.

4. Fries JF: Aging, natural death and the compression of morbidity. N Eng J Med 1980;303:130-135.

5. Kannel WB: Chapter 1: An overview of the risk factors for cardiovascular disease. IN: Kaplan NM and Stamler J (eds.): Prevention of Coronary Heart Disease. Philadelphia: W.B. Saunders, 1983.

6. Veterans Administration Cooperative Study Group on Antihypertension Agents: Effects of treatment on morbidity in hypertension. JAMA 1970;213:1143-1152.

7. Multiple Risk Factor Intervention Trial Research Group: Multiple risk factor intervention trial. JAMA 1982;248:1465-1477.

8. Hypertension Detection and Follow-up Program Cooperative Group: Five-year findings of the hypertension detection and follow-up program. JAMA 1979;242:2563-2571.

9. Farquhar JW, Maccoby N, Wood PD, et al.: Community education for cardiovascular health. Lancet 1977;1:1192-1195.

10. Lipid Research Clinical Program: The lipid research clinics coronary primary prevention trial results. JAMA 1984;251:351-364.

11. Hulley SB, Feigal D, Ireland C, et al: Systolic hypertension in the elderly program (SHEP). J Geriatrics Soc 1986;34:101-105.

12. Rose G: Strategy of prevention: Lessons from cardiovascular disease. Brit Med J 1981;282:1847-1851.

13. Veterans Administration Cooperative Study Group on Antihypertension Agents: Effects of treatment on morbidity in hypertension. Circulation 1972;45:991-1004.

14. Abramson JH and Kark SL: Community-oriented primary care: Meaning and scope. IN: Connor E and Mullen F: Community Oriented Primary Care. Washington, DC: National Academy Press, 1983.

15. Thorner RM and Remein QR: Principles and Procedures in the Evaluation of Screening for Disease. U.S. Public Health Monograph, 1961; No. 67.

16. Shapiro S: Evidence for screening for breast cancer from a randomized trial. Cancer, supplement 1977;39:2772-2782.

17. Friedman GD: Primer of Epidemiology. New York: McGraw-Hill Book Co. 1980, Chapter 14.

18. Spitzer WO (Chairman): The periodic health examination. Report of the Canadian Task Force on Periodic Health Examination. Can Med Assoc J 1979;121:1193-1254.

19. Frame PS: A critical review of adult health maintenance. J Fam Practice 1986;22:341-346.

20. American Cancer Society: Guidelines for the cancer-related check-up: Recommendations and rationale. Ca (monograph), July/August 1980.

21. Larson EB, Olsen E, Cole W, Shortell S: The relationship of health beliefs and a postcard reminder to influenza vaccination. J Fam Practice 1979;8:1207-1211.

23. American Heart Association: Coronary Risk Handbook. New York, 1973.

24. Barker W (ed.): Teaching Preventive Medicine in Primary Care. New York: Springer Publishing Co., 1983: Chapters 4, 5 and 18.

CHAPTER 3

The Methods of Clinical Prevention

Joseph Stokes III, M.D.

INTRODUCTION

Assume that you are an established primary care health professional practicing with three other partners in a single-specialty group. Mrs. M., a 44 year-old widow, whom you have not seen in your office for several years, makes an appointment to see you for a "checkup." At the time of her appointment she soon reveals that her younger sister has just had surgery for cancer of the breast and admits that her principal reason for seeking your services is for reassurance that she doesn't have cancer herself. You and your partners have recently reorganized your practice in order to be able to deliver preventive services more efficiently; you are delighted by this opportunity to comply, if possible, with her request. You also take this opportunity to encourage Mrs. M. to undergo health and risk assessment and to negotiate a health maintenance plan.

Both the organization of your practice and your approach to Mrs. M. should be guided by a clear sense of purpose. Primary care health professionals often confuse the various options that they have in approaching patients who seek their services. The approach should be responsive to the presenting problems. Most patients make initial appointments either because of symptoms caused by disease or for fear that they may be sick. Health professionals should make certain that their workup is responsive to their patient's concerns and that it is tailored to meet their needs.

If this is the patient's first visit, the initial examination may include certain base-line data, such as a resting electrocardiogram, that may prove useful when the patient comes into the emergency room at 2:00 AM with crushing chest pain. The <u>diagnostic</u> exam, under these circumstances, is expanded into a <u>base-line</u> examination.

Neither of these approaches, however, serves the purposes of the health maintenance examination, which is a periodic, proactive service that should be offered to each patient "either to maintain or improve an individual's health as contrasted to the treatment of disease" (Appendix 3.1). Health maintenance examinations are designed to check patients for some conditions on an annual basis; other checks need be performed only initially or at intervals of three to five years. Still other checks, such as flexible sigmoidoscopy, are made only once on low-risk patients at age forty (Appendices 3.3a to 3.3c).

In view of the demands being made on patients who are suffering from symptomatic illness and the difficulties in being reimbursed for preventive services by health insurance carriers, issues of efficiency are paramount. Yet, patients should not be run through "an assembly line." You know from your experience with Mrs. M. that she will demand your personal attention and that otherwise you will have little chance to impress upon her that the exam is worth her effort.

The methods of clinical prevention are as easy to define as they are difficult to implement. First, a health and risk assessment is made. This allows the health professional and patient to negotiate a health maintenance plan. This plan usually includes a set of interventions which need only be performed once, or at infrequent intervals, such as diphtheria-tetanus immunization. These procedures in turn effect health status modification. The plan also usually includes suggested changes in the patient's health behavior such as dietary change, which is defined as risk status modification. The methods are cyclical in that it is imperative for the health professional to determine if behavior change has actually taken place. Therefore, a system of tracking is essential including annual health and risk assessment according to recommended protocols in Appendices 3.3a-3.3c.

The process of health maintenance that you will recommend to Mrs. M. is comprised of three stages (see Figure 3.1). You should first persuade her to undergo health and risk assessment and you will then use this assessment to negotiate a health maintenance plan. If appropriate, you may also ask her to execute formally either an agreement or a contract. As part of the plan, and most difficult, you will try to persuade her to make changes in some of her behaviors, such as her diet, that may be required to maintain, if not improve, both her health and risk status. Finally, you will continue to assess Mrs. M. according to the recommended protocol.

HEALTH AND RISK ASSESSMENT (HRA)

The Purposes

The purpose of health assessment (Appendix 3.1) is to determine the status of the patient's health. Risk assessment is the process of obtaining the information that you need to estimate the likelihood of moving from the current level of health status to any other level of health status over a defined period of time.[1] Health maintenance usually utilizes estimates of from five to ten years. For instance, data from the Framingham Heart Study estimate risk of developing coronary heart disease over either the next six or eight years,[2] and the health risk appraisal system of the Centers for Disease Control[3] is based upon Geller Tables of age, sex and race-specific risk of death from various causes over the subsequent ten years. This latter system is, in turn, based upon the original concept of health hazard appraisal developed by Drs. Lewis Robbins and Jack Hall.[4]

THE METHODS OF CLINICAL PREVENTION   31

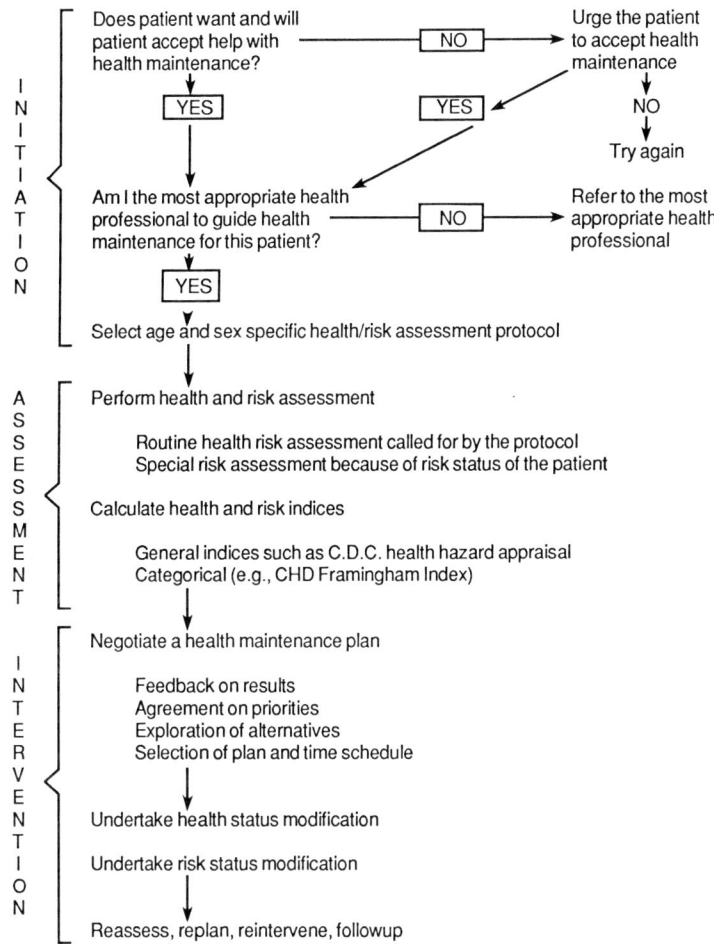

Figure 3.1. The process of clinical prevention.

DETERMINATION OF HEALTH STATUS

Subjective Assessment by the Patient

The determinants of health status are included in Table 3.1. The patient's personal assessment of health is, rightfully, at the head of the list. This is important not only because it often represents the most efficient means of obtaining a global assessment of the true status of an individual's health but also because although there may be a large discrepancy between her subjective assessment and the objective level of her function, Mrs. M. may be more likely to act upon her own perceptions than she is upon another's. Whether or not a patient receives a health service is more dependent on patient demand and health insurance coverage than it is upon whether health professionals believe that it is needed. In other words, what the patient demands, needs, and gets is not always the same.

Table 3.1
The Essential Elements of a Health Index

HEALTH STATUS	•	A global, subjective sense of well being.
	•	Objective measurement of the ability to perform valued social roles.
RISK STATUS	•	The ability to cope with physical, microbiological, and social stressors.
	•	The absence of risk of dysfunction and untimely death.

Most of the information needed to assess health status can be obtained by asking the patient to complete a self-administered health and risk assessment questionnaire. The Cornell Medical Index was one of the first of such questionnaires to be introduced to ambulatory adult medical practice and many other instruments have been developed during the last 30 years. The one currently used by the health risk appraisal system of the Centers for Disease Control (CDC) is included in Appendix 3.2. The CDC provides a computer program which analyzes the patient's responses in terms of the longevity which can be expected given the patient's health and risk status. The printout of this program for Mrs. M. is included as Appendix 3.4. Such instruments systematically obtain information unbiased by an interviewer. They also relieve health professionals of the time required to obtain the same information during an interactive interview. They are particularly useful in health maintenance where most of the information needed is unambiguous, focused and, discrete (eg, "Approximately how many miles do you drive each year in a motor vehicle?") and where efficiency is of prime importance.

They can also be computer-based using interactive software programs which make them more fun to take and much easier to analyze. Self-administered questionnaires will, of course, miss those important, non-verbal clues that can only be picked up by an astute observer during an interview. They also have limited value, at best, for open-ended questions and for those related to issues that arouse emotions such as sexual behavior. Such questionnaires are particularly useful as a means of providing patients an initial orientation to the health maintenance examintion. For instance, Mrs. M. has previously sought services only because of symptomatic illness. Despite her anxiety about breast cancer, she now needs to understand that the purposes and process of the health maintenance examination will be very different than those which are used for symptomatic illness.

Three questions are suitable to obtain the patient's self-assessment of state of health:

- "How well do you feel?";
- "How well do you feel as compared to how you felt a year ago?";
- "How well do you feel as compared with the average individual your own age and sex?

Objective Assessment by the Health Professional

Talcott Parsons[5] defined health as "the ability to perform valued social roles." There is a growing concensus that either measuring objectively, or asking patients to estimate, ability to fulfill responsibilities for themselves, their family and friends, their employer, and their communitites represents the most important index of health status. However, these roles are not easy to define precisely in terms that can be understood both by you and the patient. They also overlap and interact, and some may not apply to each patient. If this is to be a truly objective evaluation, you may want to obtain information from Mrs. M.'s family, her friends, and other peers rather than depending on her own answers to such questions as, "Do you consider the ties between you and your family to be close or distant?" Since the death of her husband a year ago, Mrs. M. has worked at a local bank. Whether or not she has been promoted and the level of her salary may be more pertinent indices of her performance than her own assessment as to how well she's doing in her job.

Any index must cope with the dilemma of weighting its various elements. If functional performance in these four roles (ie, self, family and friends, work, and community) represents the essence of health, as Parsons suggests, then the values assigned to each become critical. If such values are to be assigned, it is crucial that the weighting be done by the patient and not by the physician or nurse. Some investigators have developed research indices, the elements of which are weighted by a jury of peers,[6] but in the clinical setting, it should certainly not be done by the health professional. Obviously, if the patient aspires to rob banks, society is going to intervene, but even here, the health professional should still remain a neutral observer. The Golden Rule of Health Care is to "do unto the patient as they would have you do unto them." In the past, gaining knowledge about what the patient does or does not value has been included under the general rubric of "knowing the patient as a person." An obvious example as to how a given illness can affect two patients in different ways is to imagine the effect of laryngitis on a Met soprano, on one hand, and on a longshoreman on the other. The soprano would be temporarily totally disabled for work while the longshoreman would probably be able to carry on without even turning to a health professional for help. On the other hand, bursitis of the left shoulder may have the opposite effect.

In summary, how well patients do for themselves, for their families and friends, at work, and in their communities is the best measure of their health status. However, if their performance in these various roles is to be incorporated into a single, objective assessment, the weighting should be guided by the patient's own values.

DETERMINATION OF RISK STATUS

Ability to Cope with Stress (Adaptability)

The first step in determining risk status is to find out how well the patient can cope with stress. Ability to cope with a physical workload can be estimated from the patient's exercise tolerance. If more precise information is required, an exercise treadmill test can be carried out. The ability to cope with potential microbiological pathogens can be estimated by determining the patient's immune status and the frequency of infections. If more precision is needed, the concentration of white blood cells and circulating antibodies can be measured. Although the measurement of the patient's ability to cope with emotionally stressful events (such as the death of Mrs. M.'s husband) is of at least equal importance, it is very difficult to measure such stressors.[7] Such events cannot always be assumed to be stressful since the death of an abusive husband can be a blessing rather than a cause of grief.

The adaptive aspects of health assessment also begin to move the focus of the process from the current level of health and functional performance to prediction of the future. The most reliable means of prediction is usually to extrapolate from the past. Therefore, if Mrs. M. failed to cope effectively with the loss of her husband, this may predict trouble ahead if she looses another individual with whom she has a strong emotional tie.

Identification of Risk Factors and Remediable, Unrecognized Disease

The most important aspect of determination of risk status is to assess those factors which, although they have no immediate impact on health status, can predict the likelihood of the patient becoming sick and of not living out three score years and ten. As illustrated in Table 3.2, all of the ten leading causes of potential-years-of-life-lost (PYLL) before the age of 65 (excepting those causes during the first year of life) can be predicted by one or more risk factors, most of which are modifiable. For instance, atherosclerosis was considered by many pathologists to be an integral and inevitable aspect of aging. We now know that it is not inevitable but is due to an explicit set of causes, most of which are subject to modification. Therefore, over the last 30 years, coronary heart disease, which has ranked as the leading cause of death, is now the third ranking cause of potential-years-of-life-lost under the age of 65 in the United States. It has now become not only a highly predictable disease[8] but also a preventable disease.[9] Mrs. M. may also be advised that keeping her weight down will somewhat reduce her risk of developing cancer of the breast.[10]

Table 3.2
Rank Order of Causes of Untimely Mortality Between the Ages of 1 and 65 in the United States-1984

CAUSES	POTENTIAL YEARS OF LIFE LOST BETWEEN AGE 1 AND 65 (BY PERSONS DYING in 1984)*	ESTIMATED NUMBER OF PHYSICIAN CONTACTS MAY, 1985 (10^5)**	RANK ORDER OF IMPORTANCE OF 10 RISK FACTORS
Unintentional injuries	2,308,000	54	1. Accident-risk behavior 2. Alcohol abuse
Cancer	1,803,000	13	1. Cigarette smoking 2. Obesity 3. Alcohol abuse
Heart disease	1,563,000	63	1. Dyslipidemia 2. Hypertension 3. Cigarette smoking 4. Hyperglycemia 5. Obesity 6. Alcohol abuse 7. Exercise intolerance
Suicide and homicide	1,247,000	--	1. Alcohol abuse
Stroke	266,000	8	1. Hypertension 2. Dyslipidemia 3. Hyperglycemia 4. Cigarette smoking 5. Obesity 6. Alcohol abuse
Cirrhosis	233,000	1	1. Alcohol abuse
Pneumonia	163,000	14	1. Alcohol abuse 2. Immunization failure
Chronic obstructive lung disease	123,000	3	1. Cigarette smoking
Diabetes	119,000	32	1. Hyperglycemia 2. Obesity

* Data from MMWR 35:P105, February 21, 1986.
** Data from IMS American National Disease and Therapeutic. Index, Monthly Report, March 1985.

The logic of risk assessment can be developed within one of several conceptual models of causation. The traditional epidemiologic model is most useful in understanding the pathogenesis of infectious and other diseases where a single environmental agent represents a cause. This model envisions an environmental reservoir of such an agent reaching a susceptible host by means of either a passive vehicle or an active insect vector. Other models have been used for accident control where several environmental factors play key roles.[11] However, the model that works best for cardiovascular disease, cancer, and other chronic multifactorial diseases was first described by McKeown[12] as an extension of the nature:nurture concept of pathogenesis. As illustrated in Figure 3.2, this model assumes that both health and disease can be ascribed to inheritance and the various elements of the physical, biological, and social environment over which individuals have little control. Individuals cope with these relatively fixed (ie, nonmodifiable) factors through health behaviors. These not only effect the primary prevention of disease but also include self-care of disease, health care-seeking behavior, and the adherence by the patient to drug and other regimens prescribed by professionals, all of which play important roles in secondary prevention.

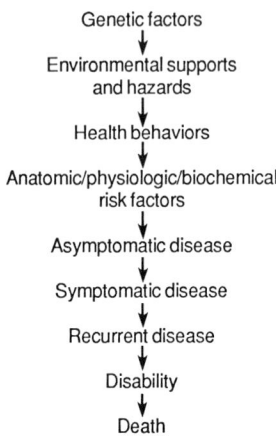

Figure 3.2. The McKeown model of health and disease.

Genetic and environmental factors and both supportive and destructive health behaviors may all then be reflected in various anatomic (eg, obesity), physiologic (eg, blood pressure) and biochemical (eg, serum cholesterol) conditions that also play important causal roles (Table 3.3). Certain diseases, including that which is the focus of Mrs. M.'s concern, have latent periods between the time that they first develop and the time when they first cause signs sufficient to permit their identification by means of screening procedures. They can be treated more effectively during this time than is possible after symptoms develop. The most important of these asymptomatic, remediable conditions and diseases of adults are listed in Table 3.4.

Table 3.3
Anatomic, Physiologic, and Biochemical Risk Factors for Adults

FACTOR	METHOD OF MEASUREMENT
Obesity	1. Body mass index (Weight/Height^2) 2. Skin fold thickness 3. Waist:hip ratio
Systemic arterial blood pressure	1. Resting 2. In response to stress 3. 24-hour monitoring
Lung function	1. Vital capacity 2. Forced expiratory volume in 1 second (FEV 1) 3. Carbon monoxide content of expired air (PPM)
Serum lipids and sterols	1. Total cholesterol (TC) 2. High density lipoprotein Cholesterol (HDL-C) 3. Triglycerides (TG)
Blood sugar	1. Fasting 2. Random 3. Glycosolated hemoglobin (A1 Hgb)
Cardiac	Electrocardiographic measurement of: 1. Heart rate (HR) 2. Cardiac rhythm 3. Pattern of left ventricular hypertrophy 4. Evidence of prior myocardial infarction
Resistance to infection	1. White blood count and differential 2. Circulating antibodies 3. T-Cell function

Table 3.4
The Major Asymptomatic Remediable Diseases of Adults

DISEASE	PRIMARY SCREENING	SECONDARY SCREENING
Blood loss anemia	Hemoglobin/hematocrit	CBC and red cell indices
Breast cancer	Breast exam X-ray mammography	Excisional biopsy
Cancer of cervix	Pap smear	Biopsy
Cirrhosis	Serum gamma glutamyl Transpeptidase	Full battery of liver function tests
Colo-rectal cancer	Hemoccult	Endoscopy Barium enema
Deafness	Screening audiometry	Complete audiometry
Glaucoma	Ophthalmoscopic exam and tonometry	Visual fields
Hypertension	Blood pressure	
Osteoporosis	Personal and family history	X-ray bone density
Presbyopia	Visual acuity	
Syphilis	Serologic test for syphilis (VDRL)	Treponema pallidum-specific antibody
Testicular cancer	Exam of scrotum	
Tuberculosis	Tuberculin testing (PPD)	Chest X-ray
Urinary tract infection	Quantitative urine	

In addition, some symptomatic diseases have emerged that should alert the primary care health professional to take action to prevent their recurrence. For example, it has been shown that drugs that block the beta adrenergic receptors of the heart can prevent a recurrence of myocardial infarction and sudden death.[13] Patients who have had cancer of the skin, breast, or colon are at higher risk for recurrence of these cancers than are those who have been cancer free.[14] Indeed, most patients who have had one cancer are probably more prone to develop another, and the awareness of this fact should alert both patient and health professional.

Methods of Health and Risk Assessment (HRA)

SELECTION OF AGE-SEX RISK SPECIFIC PROTOCOLS

The protocols that guide the health and risk assessment of men and women in the three age groups from adolescence to old age are listed in Appendix 3.3a-3.3c. These protocols have been modified from those suggested by Breslow and Somers[15] in the classic article which appeared in 1977 and stemmed from a task force report of the Conference on Preventive Medicine sponsored by the National Institutes of Health and the American College of Preventive Medicine in 1975. More extensive analysis has also been performed by the Canadian Task Force on the periodic health examination which was reported initially in 1979[16] and has subsequently updated in 1984.[17] These reports define and apply strict rules of evidence to guide the recommendations. They have also stimulated others such as the American Cancer Society,[18] the American College of Physicians,[19] and the American Medical Association[20] to develop similar guidelines. The criteria used by the Canadian (and subsequently by the U.S.) Task Force have been:

- The quality of scientific evidence regarding the efficacy of either primary and secondary prevention;
- The degree to which the disease or condition can cause serious morbidity and untimely death; and
- The sensitivity, specificity, cost, safety and acceptability of screening procedure proposed.

In addition, concern should be directed as to whether or not a positive screening test (such as the identification of hypertension) may inappropriately label an individual as sick and encourage that person to begin to play the sick role.[22]

Despite the plethora of expert reports, every protocol must be adapted to the style of the practice where it is to be applied. In addition, both the procedures used to identify asymptomatic, remediable disease and the interventions made to improve health status should be adjusted according to the patient's individual risk status. For example, young women who became sexually active early and continue to engage in sex with many partners should have cervical cytologic exams every year while older women with only one sexual partner and who have had three or more negative cervical cytologies in the past need only be retested at five-year intervals. Annual influenza immunization should be reserved for those patients 65 or over and others at high risk.

THE PROCESS OF HEALTH AND RISK ASSESSMENT (HRA)

The process of HRA is analogous to the evaluation of a patient who has a symptomatic illness. It begins with obtaining a medical history, which, as indicated above, is most efficiently done by means of a self-administered questionnaire. The physical examination of the HRA is <u>always</u> selective and usually carried out by a nurse practitioner or a physician's assistant. The laboratory and special procedures should also be carefully selected according to age and sex-specific protocols and other indices of special risk (Appendices 3.3a-3.3c). Although the analysis of this information usually does not result in any specific diagnoses, a problem list should be generated.

The problem list includes the goals that the health professional would like to achieve. The list thus serves as the basis for negotiation with the patient regarding a health maintenance plan (HMP) and a health maintenance agreement which almost invariably will include one or more changes in health behavior. The goals of the HMP should focus particularly upon modification of the anatomic-physiologic and biochemical pathogenic factors listed in Table 3.3. First, certain abnormalities found at the time of HRA will need to be studied further in order to establish the presence of remediable disease (e.g., Table 3.4). Next come those interventions designed to modify health status by means of a simple, single intervention such as immunization or eyeglasses. Finally, the most difficult interventions are those that attempt to modify one or more health behaviors such as diet which are designed to improve the patient's risk status but which may take months or years to achieve.

As mentioned above, efficiency can be enhanced by computer-based information, storage, and retrieval systems which can also be used to help with the process of health and risk appraisal such as that which has been developed by the Centers for Disease Control. Health professionals should also participate in analysis of the data and in negotiating the health maintenance plan. It is essential that the physician, nurse, and other providers who perform the health and risk assessment convey to the patient that they place a high priority on health maintenance services and that they reinforce these recommendations by modeling optimal health behaviors themselves.

DEVELOPMENT OF THE HEALTH MAINTENANCE PLAN

A copy of Mrs. M.'s CDC/HRA is included as Appendix 3.4 which will serve as the basis for your recommendations to her in her health maintenance plan. Both timing and priorities are important. One can build confidence by proposing that the patient attempt a relatively easy task first, particularly if it is one that makes the patient feel better. For example, as is the case with most of her peers, Mrs. M. is overweight. It should be possible for her to lose approximately one pound each week over the next 20 weeks in order to reach her optimum weight. However, it may be wiser to begin with an exercise program rather than with reducing her caloric intake since the exercise program is easier to accomplish and will probably make her feel better. Explain your rationale as you negotiate the health maintenance plan with the patient. This will let the patient understand your logic. This negotiating process will also provide you with a better idea of the patient's values and priorities.

RISK STATUS (HEALTH BEHAVIOR) MODIFICATION

As stated above, the greatest challenge of clinical health maintenance is to effect risk factor modification. Difficult though the task may be, health professionals are far more effective than they may realize in modifying the patient's behavior. They are also in the unique position of being able to identify the "teachable moment," ie, the time that the patient finally realizes that a change in health behavior is necessary. Mrs. M. is an excellent example in that the occurrence in her sister of carcinoma of the breast has increased her willingness to comply with a mammographic exam.

Although the behavioral methods that are used will be discussed in greater detail in Chapter 5, the following guidelines are particularly important for the physician/nurse to keep in mind:

- <u>Make sure that the patient is aware of your objectives.</u> If you are modifying an anatomic, physiologic or biochemical factor such as body weight, express your goal in precise, quantitative terms that the patient can easily understand.
- <u>Explain the reasons for your suggesting these goals.</u> As explained above under the negotiation of the health maintenance plan, it is critical that the rational basis for the goals are clear.
- <u>Be certain that the patient has access to the various means of achieving these goals.</u> It is manifestly ineffective to suggest that Mrs. M. join a smoking withdrawal group if none is available in the community.
- <u>Employ motivational methods as often as possible.</u> Remember that fear, love, and money can go a long way towards modifying behaviors. There is nothing wrong with dramatizing the various dire consequences of continued, self-destructive behavior such as cigarette smoking. If you have established good rapport with your patient, it may be effective for you to suggest that you, yourself, would be very pleased to have Mrs. M. stop smoking since patients generally do wish to please those health professionals whose counsel they have sought.

  Even more important, try to use the "exchange system" whereby patients can be rewarded for making a positive change in their life style. Remember that the ultimate reward for making a change in behavior is that nothing happens many years hence. Indeed, it is remarkable that so many patients actually do make such changes in order to achieve such a long-deferred reward. Therefore, try to devise other more immediate rewards such as returning money placed in escrow. Motivation is one of the biggest challenges to clinical health maintenance.[22]

- **Start with easy tasks** and defer the most difficult. This will allow the patient to build confidence that they can modify their behavior. For instance, you would begin by encouraging Mrs. M. to develop an exercise program and would not recommend that she stop smoking until she has achieved such a goal.
- **Monitor patients frequently during the early phases of the program.** This will allow you to modify the patient's health maintenance program promptly if difficulties are encountered.
- **Don't depend exclusively on a cognitive approach.** Merely providing the patient with the facts is rarely sufficient to change an entrenched health behavior.
- **Don't suggest any behavior that you don't model yourself.** What you do will speak so loudly that patients won't hear what you say.

SPECIAL CONSIDERATIONS

Although the modification of health behavior will be most effective if it is accomplished during adolescence and early adulthood, adolescents loathe advice from parents, health professionals, and other authority figures. During both adolescence and early adulthood the consequences of suboptimal health behavior are so remote that their effects are heavily discounted by young patients, who imagine that if they should eventually succumb to one or another risk-related disease, some miracle of therapeutic medicine will have been developed by that time which can "bail them out."

Another general rule is that those patients who believe they are in control of their lives are usually more willing to modify their health behaviors. This is often referred to as the "locus of control." In essence, such individuals are experienced in planning ahead and have a sense of investment in the future. They consider their health to be a capital asset and they are often willing to give up some cherished behaviors such as cigarette smoking in order to avoid a future, but as yet unfelt, event. Unfortunately, low income populations usually do not have such a proactive philosophy and may be trapped in the present. They may be discouraged and apprehensive about the future. It may be for these reasons that, in general, the worst risk profiles are currently among those of lowest socioeconomic status.[23]

Clinical health maintenance can be practiced in a variety of settings (Table 3.5). Each has advantages and disadvantages. The freestanding clinic can be designed and staffed for maximum efficiency and is not burdened by overhead costs that are often carried by clinics at other sites. However, it labors under the serious disadvantages of discontinuity with those services that are usually required for modifying health behavior and for the diagnosis and treatment of asymptomatic, remediable disease. Many traditional occupational health services have recently expanded to include preventive services, but most small businesses cannot afford separate work-site programs. These also share with the free-standing clinics the problem of discontinuity. In addition, employees may be suspicious that such programs are introduced primarily to increase productivity and to decrease absenteeism and the cost of health insurance rather than to improve the employee's health. Fortunately, the two objectives are fully compatible with each other.

Table 3.5
Comparison of Sites for Health Maintenance Services

SITE	ADVANTAGES	DISADVANTAGES
Free-standing	Efficiency	Lack of linkage for referral
Work	Access to patients (Employees)	(Same as free-standing)
		Role conflicts
Primary care	Close linkage for referral and continuity of care	Competition for time and other resources with symptomatic patients
	Opportunistic services at time of illness services	

The primary care setting may be somewhat less efficient in the delivery of a discrete package of preventive services, but efficiency can be increased by integrating such services into other types of primary health care. It certainly has the clear advantage of close linkage for referral. However, if the program is part of a secondary or tertiary hospital, it must contend with the problem of competition for time and other resources with symptomatic patients. Health professionals can hardly be blamed for neglecting preventive services to respond to the needs of sick patients.

As mentioned above, efficiency is important and can be enhanced by computer-based information storage and retrieval systems which can be used to help with the process of health and risk appraisals. Health professionals should also participate in analysis of the data and in negotiating the health maintenance plan. It is essential that the physician, nurse, and other providers who perform health risk assessment give the patient the idea that they place a high priority on these health maintenance services and that they reinforce these recommendations by modeling optimum health behaviors themselves. What's more, preventive services can be "piggybacked" onto diagnostic and therapeutic services performed at ambulatory care settings.[24]

SUMMARY

Clinical health maintenance is an essential aspect of primary care. It is practiced by means of periodic examinations consisting of an initial health and risk assessment followed by annual assessment guided by specific protocols. It can be practiced in a variety of settings, each of which has specific advantages and disadvantages. The emphasis should be upon efficiency, and a clear distinction should be made between the periodic examination and that which is performed for the initial, baseline assessment of a new patient and most certainly from that which is done because of symptomatic illness. Health and risk assessment and health maintenance planning can be performed with precision and relative ease providing one has a cooperative patient. The most difficult aspect of health maintenance is effecting behavior change in order to modify the critical, anatomic, physiologic and biochemical factors that are predictive of serious morbidity and untimely death.

REFERENCES:

1. Fanshel S, Bush JW: A health status index and its applications to health services outcomes. Operations Res 1970;18:1021-1066.

2. Abbott RD, Garrison RJ, Wilson PWF, Castelli WP: Coronary heart disease risk: The importance of joint relationships among cholesterol levels in individual lipoprotein classes. Preventive Med 1982;11:131-141.

3. Wagner EH, Beery WL, Schoenbach VJ, Graham RM: An assessment of health hazard/health risk appraisal. Amer J Public Health 1982; 72:347-352.

4. Hall JH, Zwemer JD: Prospective Medicine (ed. 2). Indianapolis: Methodist Hospital of Indiana, Dept. of Medical Education, 1979.

5. Parsons T: Definitions of Health and Illness in Light of American Values and Social Structure (ed. 2). Glencoe, NY: Free Press, 1948.

6. Kaplan RM, Bush JW, Berry CC: Health Status Index: Category rating versus magnitude estimation for measuring levels of well-being. Med Care 1979;5:501-523.

7. Haynes SG, Levine S, Scotch NA, et al: The relationship of psychosocial factors to coronary heart disease in the Framingham Study. Amer J Epidem 1978;107:362-383.

8. Shurtleff D: Some Characteristics Related to the Incidence of Cardiovascular Disease and Death: The Framingham Study. Kanne WB and Gordon T (eds.). Washington, DC: Government Printing Office, February 1974.

9. Blackburn H: Public policy and dietary recommendations to reduce population levels of blood cholesterol. Amer J Preventive Med 1985; 1:3-11.

10. Gray GE, Pike MC, Henderson BE: Breast cancer incidence and mortality rates in different countries in relation to known risk factors and dietary practices. Brit J Cancer 1979;39:1-7.

11. Haddon W Jr.: A note concerning accident theory and research with special reference to motor vehicle accidents. Ann NY Adac Sci 1963; 107:635-646.

12. McKeown T, Lowe CR: An Introduction to Social Medicine (ed. 2). Oxford: Blackwell Scientific Publications, 1974.

13. Beta Blocker Heart Attack Study Group: The Beta Blocker Heart Attack Trial. JAMA 1981;246:2073.

14. Fraumeni JR Jr.: Persons at High Risk of Cancer: An Approach to Cancer Etiology and Control. New York: Academic Press Inc., 1975.

15. Breslow L and Somers AR: The lifetime health monitoring program: A practical approach to preventive medicine. N Eng J Med 1977;206: 601-608.

16. Canadian Task Force on the Periodic Health Examination: The periodic health examination. Can Med Assoc J 1979;121:1193-1254.

17. Canadian Task Force on the Periodic Health Examination: The periodic health examination, 1984 update. Can Med Assoc J 1984;130:1278-1285.

18. American Cancer Society: Mammography guidelines 1983: Background statement and update of cancer-related check-up guidelines breast cancer detection in asymptomatic women, age 40 to 49. Cancer 1983; 33:255.

19. Medical Practice Committee, American College of Physicians: Periodic health examintion: A guide for designing individualized preventive health care in the asymptomatic patient. Ann Internal Med 1981;95: 729-732.

20. Council on Scientific Affairs, Division of Scientific Activities, American Medical Association: Medical evaluations of healthy persons. JAMA 1983;249:1626-1633.

21. Haynes RB, Sackett DL, Taylor DW, Gibson ES, Johnson AL: Increased absenteeism from work after detection and labeling of hypertensive patients. N Eng J Med 1978;14:299,741-744.

22. Stokes J III: Why not rate health and life insurance premiums by risks? N Eng J Med 1983;308:393-395.

23. Syme L, Oakes TW, Friedman GD et al.: Social class and racial differences in blood pressure. Amer J Pub Health 1974;64:619-620.

24. Logsdon DN, Rosen MA, Demak MM: The INSURE Project on lifecycle preventive health services. Public Health Reports 1982;97:308-317.

Appendix 3.1
Glossary of Terms and Concepts Related to Clinical Preventive Medicine

GENERAL CONCEPTS

Health. A state characterized by anatomic integrity; ability to perform personally valued family, work, and community roles; ability to deal with physical, biological, and social stress; a feeling of well-being; freedom from the risk of disease and untimely death. It is best measured by determining health status and risk status.

Determinants of health. Those factors that have a significant effect on health. Such factors are most conveniently classified as those which are genetic, environmental (including the physical, biological and social environment), behavioral (including diet, exercise, sleep, cigarette smoking, use of alcohol and other mind-altering drugs, motor vehicle driving and other accident-risk behavior), and access to preventive, diagnostic, therapeutic, and rehabilitative health services.

Health behavior. Any behavior that has a significant impact on health.

Health hazard. Any environmental factor known to represent a significant risk to health.

Health maintenance. Any proactive intervention, the purpose of which is either to maintain or improve an individual's health as contrasted with the treatment of disease.

Primary care. Primary care is first contact care that provides the patient's entry into the health care system. The primary care provider 1) evaluates the patient's total health needs, provides personal medical care within one or more fields of medicine, and when indicated, refers the patient to appropriate sources of care while preserving the continuity of the care; 2) assumes responsibility for the patient's comprehensive and continuous health care, and acts, where appropriate, as the leader or coordinator of a team of health care providers; and 3) accepts responsibility for the patient's total health care (preventive, diagnostic, curative, and rehabilitative) within the context of his (or her) environment, including the community and the family or comparable social unit.

Screening. The process of identifying individuals with one or more remediable, asymptomatic disease or risk factor in a defined population group.

Risk factor. Any factor associated with the occurrence of disease and which is suspected of being causally related.

LEVELS OF PREVENTION

Primary prevention. Any intervention, the purpose of which is to reduce the risk of occurrence of disease.

Secondary prevention. Any intervention, the purpose of which is either to 1) detect asymptomatic, remediable disease; or 2) reduce the risk of recurrence of disease.

Prevention in clinical medicine. Any intervention in the care of an individual with a recognized disease or limiting condition which has the purpose of 1) optimizing the health status of the individual in spite of recognized disease or limiting condition; 2) anticipating and avoiding (or minimizing the likelihood of) the occurrence of complications either of the disease or of the diagnostic or therapeutic measures contemplated; or 3) reducing functional impairment which may accompany or result from a disease state or limiting condition.

From: Stokes J III, Noren J, Shindell S: Definition of terms and concepts applicable to clinical preventive medicine. Journal of Community Health, Fall 1982;8(1):39-40. Reprinted by permission.

Appendix 3.1 (Cont'd.)
Glossary of Terms and Concepts Related to Clinical Preventive Medicine

CLINICAL PREVENTION

Clinical preventive medicine. Those personal health services, provided within the context of clinical medicine, the purpose of which is to maintain health and reduce the risk of disease and untimely death.

Health status. An estimate of the state of an individual's health derived from one or more anatomic, functional, adaptive, and subjective indices.

Risk status. An estimate of the state of an individual's risk determined from data on inheritance, environmental exposures, health habits, and by identifying unrecognized, asymptomatic conditions and diseases known to increase the risk of illness and untimely death.

Health and risk assessment. The process of obtaining the information needed to determine an individual's health and risk status. These data are obtained by means of self-administered questionnaires and interviews as well as from physical and laboratory examinations.

Health maintenance plan. An integrated set of recommendations defining what should be done in order to maintain or improve an individual's health. The plan should be developed as a cooperative effort of the individual and those responsible for his or her primary health care. It should set specific objectives to be achieved after a specified period of time and should also include plans for periodic reassessment.

Health maintenance agreement. An agreement negotiated with the patient by one or more responsible health professionals, the purpose of which is both to clarify and implement the Health Maintenance Plan.

Health status modification. Those interventions such as immunizations and the provision of eyeglasses and hearing aids performed by health professionals, the purpose of which is to maintain or improve current health status.

Risk status modification. Those interventions, the purpose of which is to reduce the risk of future disease and untimely death and to improve future health status.

Health and risk reassessment. The process of obtaining the information from an individual needed to determine whether or not the objectives of the Health Maintenance Plan have been achieved and to modify the Plan because of changes in that individual's health and risk status.

From: Stokes J III, Noren J, Shindell S: Definition of terms and concepts applicable to clinical preventive medicine. Journal of Community Health, Fall 1982;8(1):39-40. Reprinted by permission.

Appendix 3.2
Health Risk Appraisal.

Health Risk Appraisal is a promising health education tool that is still in the early stages of development. It is designed to show how your individual lifestyle affects your chances of avoiding the most common causes of death for a person of your age, race and sex. It also shows how much you can improve your chances by changing your harmful habits. (This particular version is not very useful for persons under 25 or over 60 years old and for persons who have had a heart attack or other serious medical problem.)

IMPORTANT: To assure protection of your privacy, do NOT put your name on this form. Make sure that you put your Health Risk Appraisal "coupon" in your wallet or other safe place and insure that the number matches the number on this form. You must present your coupon to get your computer results.

PARTICIPANT NUMBER _____ 1-6

PLEASE ENTER YOUR ANSWERS IN THE EMPTY BOXES (use numbers only)

1. SEX — [1] Male [2] Female — 7

2. RACE/ORIGIN — [1] White (non-Hispanic origin) [2] Black (non-Hispanic origin) [3] Hispanic [4] Asian or Pacific Islander [5] American Indian or Alaskan Native [6] Not sure — 8

3. AGE (At Last Birthday) — Years Old — 9-10

4. HEIGHT (Without Shoes) — Example: 5 foot, 7½ inches = [5] [0][8] " (No Fractions) — 11-13

5. WEIGHT (Without Shoes) — Pounds — 14-16

6. TOBACCO — [1] Smoker [2] Ex-Smoker [3] Never Smoked — 17

(Smokers and Ex-smokers) Enter average number smoked per day in the last five years (ex-smokers should use the last five years before quitting.)
- Cigarettes Per Day — 18-19
- Pipes/Cigars Per Day (Smoke Inhaled) — 20-21
- Pipes/Cigars Per Day (Smoke Not Inhaled) — 22-23

(Ex-smokers only) Enter Number of Years Stopped Smoking (Note: Enter 1 for less than one year) — 24-25

7. ALCOHOL — [1] Drinker [2] Ex-Drinker (Stopped) [3] Non-Drinker (or drinks less than one drink per week) — 26

If you drink alcohol, enter the average number of drinks per week:
- Bottles of beer per week — 27-28
- Glasses of wine per week — 29-30
- Mixed drinks or shots of liquor per week — 31-32

8. DRUGS/MEDICATION How often do you use drugs or medication which affect your mood or help you to relax? [1] Almost every day [2] Sometimes [3] Rarely or Never — 33

9. MILES Per Year as a driver of a motor vehicle and/or passenger of an automobile (10,000 = average) Thousands of miles — 0 0 0 34-38

10. SEAT BELT USE (percent of time used) Example: about half the time = [5][0] — % 39-41

11. PHYSICAL ACTIVITY LEVEL
- [1] Level 1 - little or no physical activity
- [2] Level 2 - occasional physical activity
- [3] Level 3 - regular physical activity at least 3 times per week

NOTE: Physical activity includes work and leisure activities that require sustained physical exertion such as walking briskly, running, lifting and carrying. — 42

12. Did either of your parents die of a heart attack before age 60? [1] Yes, One of them [2] Yes, Both of them [3] No [4] Not sure — 43

13. Did your mother, father, sister or brother have diabetes? [1] Yes [2] No [3] Not sure — 44

14. Do YOU have diabetes? [1] Yes, not controlled [2] Yes, controlled [3] No [4] Not sure — 45

15. Rectal problems (other than piles or hemorrhoids). Have you had:
- Rectal Growth? [1] Yes [2] No [3] Not sure — 46
- Rectal Bleeding? [1] Yes [2] No [3] Not sure — 47
- Annual Rectal Exam? [1] Yes [2] No [3] Not sure — 48

CDC 90.4 4-82

(Continued on Other Side)

From: Sachs JS et al: Reliability of the Health Hazard Appraisal. American Journal of Public Health, 1981;70:730-732. Form originally by Centers for Disease Control, Atlanta, GA. Reprinted by permission.

Appendix 3.2 (Cont'd.)
Health Risk Appraisal.

16. Has your physician ever said you have Chronic Bronchitis or Emphysema? ☐1 Yes ☐2 No ☐3 Not sure ☐ 49

17. Blood Pressure (If known — otherwise leave blank) Systolic (High Number) ☐☐☐ 50-52
    Diastolic (Low Number) ☐☐☐ 53-55

18. Fasting Cholesterol Level (If known — otherwise leave blank) MG/DL ☐☐☐ 56-58

19. Considering your age, how would you describe your overall physical health?
    ☐1 Excellent ☐2 Good ☐3 Fair ☐4 Poor ☐ 59

20. In general not satisfied are you with your life?
    ☐1 Mostly Satisfied ☐2 Partly Satisfied ☐3 Mostly Disappointed ☐4 Not Sure ☐ 60

21. In general how strong are your social ties with your family and friends?
    ☐1 Very strong ☐2 About Average ☐3 Weaker than average ☐4 Not sure ☐ 61

22. How many hours of sleep do you usually get at night?
    ☐1 6 hours or less ☐2 7 hours ☐3 8 hours ☐4 9 hours or more ☐ 62

23. Have you suffered a serious personal loss or misfortune in the Past Year? (For example, a job loss, disability, divorce, separation, jail term, or the death of a close person)
    ☐1 Yes, one serious loss ☐2 Yes, Two or More serious losses ☐3 No ☐ 63

24. How often in the Past Year did you witness or become involved in a violent or potentially violent argument?
    ☐1 4 or more times ☐2 2 or 3 times ☐3 Once or never ☐4 Not sure ☐ 64

25. How many of the following things do you usually do?
    • Hitch-hike or pick up hitch-hikers • Criticize or argue with strangers
    • Carry a gun or knife for protection • Live or work at night in a high-crime area
    • Keep a gun at home for protection • Seek entertainment at night in high-crime areas or bars
    ☐1 3 or more ☐2 1 or 2 ☐3 None ☐4 Not sure ☐ 65

26. Have you had a hysterectomy? (Women only) ☐1 Yes ☐2 No ☐3 Not sure ☐ 66

27. How often do you have Pap Smear? (Women only)
    ☐1 At least once per year ☐2 At least once every 3 years ☐3 More than 3 years apart
    ☐4 Have never had one ☐5 Not sure ☐6 Not applicable ☐ 67

28. Was your last Pap Smear Normal? (Women only) ☐1 Yes ☐2 No ☐3 Not sure ☐4 Not applicable ☐ 68

29. Did your mother, sister or daughter have breast cancer? (Women only) ☐1 Yes ☐2 No ☐3 Not sure ☐ 69

30. How often do you examine your breasts for lumps? (Women only)
    ☐1 Monthly ☐2 Once every few months ☐3 Rarely or never ☐ 70

31. Have you ever completed a computerized Health Risk Appraisal Questionnaire like this one?
    ☐1 Yes ☐2 No ☐3 Not sure ☐ 71

32. Current Marital Status ☐1 Single (Never married) ☐2 Married ☐3 Separated
    ☐4 Widowed ☐5 Divorced ☐6 Other ☐ 72

33. Schooling completed (One choice only) ☐1 Did Not graduate from high school ☐2 High School
    ☐3 Some College ☐4 College or Professional Degree ☐ 73

34. Employment Status ☐1 Employed ☐2 Unemployed
    ☐3 Homemaker, Volunteer, or Student ☐4 Retired, Other ☐ 74

35. Type of occupation (SKIP IF NOT APPLICABLE)
    ☐1 Professional, Technical, Manager, Official or Proprietor ☐2 Clerical or Sales
    ☐3 Craftsman, Foreman or Operative ☐4 Service or Laborer ☐ 75

36. County of Current Residence (SKIP IF NOT KNOWN)
    [1][2][1] FULTON   [0][8][9] DEKALB
    [0][6][7] COBB   [0][6][3] CLAYTON
    [1][3][5] GWINNETT [0][5][9] CLARK   [9][9][9] Other [☐☐☐] 76-78

37. State of Current Residence [1][3] GEORGIA [9][9] Other [☐☐] 79-80)

From: Sachs JS et al: Reliability of the Health Hazard Appraisal. American Journal of Public Health, 1981;70:730-732. Form originally by Centers for Disease Control, Atlanta, GA. Reprinted by permission.

Appendix 3.3a
Preventive Services for the Young Adult (17-35 Years)

I. OBJECTIVES

- To foster an attitude of acceptance of full responsibility for health commensurate with ability
- To maintain immunization status regarding selected infectious diseases
- To reinforce good health habits and health maintenance behavior particularly in the prevention of atherosclerosis, hypertension and preventable cancers
- To provide information of family planning and birth control

II. PREVENTIVE SERVICES RECOMMENDED FREQUENCY

A. Self-administered health and risk questionnaire

• Long form	At initial exam and every five years
• Short form	Annual exam

B. Physical examination

• Height	Initial exam only
• Weight	Annual exam
• Blood pressure x2	Annual exam
• Pelvic examination and cervical cytology (women only)	Annual exam for three years and if negative every five years thereafter (low risk) Annual (high risk)
• Gonococcal cervical culture	Annual (high risk)

C. Laboratory examination

- Blood

Hematocrit	Annual exam
Serum total and HDL cholesterol	Initial exam and every five years thereafter
Serologic test for syphilis	Initial exam and every five years thereafter
Random blood sugar	Initial exam and every five years thereafter
• Urine culture (women only)	Initial exam and every three years thereafter

From: Modified from Breslow L, Somers AR: The lifetime health monitoring program: A practical approach to preventive medicine. New England Journal of Medicine, 1977;296:601-608.

Appendix 3.3a (Cont'd.)
Preventive Services for the Young Adult (17-35 Years)

- D. Testing
  - Visual acuity — Initial exam and every five years thereafter
  - Screen audiometry — Initial exam and every five years thereafter
  - Tuberculin testing — Initial exam and every five years thereafter

- E. Immunizations
  - Bivalent diphtheria-tetanus booster — Every ten years
  - Rubella immunization (women only) — Initial exam (if not previously performed)

- F. Counseling — Initial exam and every five years thereafter
  - Nutrition
  - Exercise
  - Smoking
  - Drugs and alcohol
  - Accident prevention
  - Self-examination of the breast (women only)
  - Self-examination of the genitalia (men only)
  - Family planning
  - Occupational counseling

From: Modified from Breslow L, Somers AR: The lifetime health monitoring program: A practical approach to preventive medicine. New England Journal of Medicine, 1977;296:601-608.

Appendix 3.3b
Preventive Services for the Middle-Aged Adult (36-64 Years)

I. OBJECTIVES

- To foster an attitude of acceptance of full responsibility for health commensurate with ability
- To maintain immunization status regarding selected infectious diseases
- To reinforce good health habits and health maintenance behavior particularly in the prevention of atherosclerosis, hypertension, and preventable cancers
- To prepare for retirement

II. PREVENTIVE SERVICES · RECOMMENDED FREQUENCY

A. Self-administered health and risk questionnaire

- Long form — At initial exam and every five years
- Short form — Annual exam

B. Physical examination

- Height — Initial exam only
- Weight — Annual exam
- Blood pressure x2 — Annual exam
- Rectal examination (men only) — Initial exam and every three years
- Hemoccult testing x3 — Annual exam
- Pelvic and rectal exam and cervical cytology (women only) — Initially and every five years (low risk) / Annually (high risk)
- Flexible sigmoidoscopy — Once at age 40 (high risk)

C. Laboratory examination

- Blood

Hematocrit	Initially and annually
T-cholesterol and HDL-cholesterol	Initial exam and every five years
Serologic test for syphilis	Initial exam and every five years

From: Modified from Breslow L, Somers AR: The lifetime health monitoring program: A practical approach to preventive medicine. New England Journal of Medicine, 1977;296:601-608.

Appendix 3.3b (Cont'd.)
Preventive Services for the Middle-Aged Adult (36-64 Years)

- D. Testing
    - Eyes

Visual acuity	Initial exam and every two years
Tonometry	Initially and annually

    - Screening audiometry — Initial exam and every five years
    - Tuberculin testing — Initial exam and every five years
    - Mammography (women only) — Beginning at age 50 and two years thereafter (low risk) Initial exam at 35 and every year thereafter (high risk)

- E. Immunizations
    - Bivalent diphtheria-tetanus Booster — Every ten years
    - Pneumococcal immunization — Once only, high risk only

- F. Counselling
    - Nutrition
    - Exercise
    - Smoking
    - Drugs and alcohol
    - Accident prevention
    - Self-examination of the breast (women only)
    - Self-examination of the genitalia (men only)
    - Family planning
    - Occupational counselling
    - Preparation for retirement

From: Modified from Breslow L, Somers AR: The lifetime health monitoring program: A practical approach to preventive medicine. New England Journal of Medicine, 1977;296:601-608.

Appendix 3.3c
Preventive Services for the Older Adult (65 Years and Older)

I. OBJECTIVES

- To identify asymptomatic, remediable defects prior to irreversible damage
- Retirement counselling

II. PREVENTIVE SERVICES   RECOMMENDED FREQUENCY

A. Self-administered health and risk Questionnaire

- Long form   At initial exam and every five years
- Short form   Annual exam

B. Physical examination

- Height   Initial exam only
- Weight   Annual exam
- Blood pressure x2   Annual exam
- Rectal examination (men only)   Initial exam and every three years
- Hemoccult testing x3   Annual exam
- Pelvic and rectal exam and cervical cytology (women only)   Initially and every five years (low risk) Annually (high risk)

C. Laboratory examination

- Blood

     Hematocrit   Initially and annually

D. Testing

- Eyes

     Visual acuity   Initially and annually
     Tonometry   Initially and annually

- Screening audiometry   Initially and annually

- Mammography (women only)   Initially and every two years (low risk) Initially and annually (high risk)

From: Modified from Breslow L, Somers AR: The lifetime health monitoring program: A practical approach to preventive medicine. New England Journal of Medicine, 1977;296:601-608.

Appendix 3.3c (Cont'd)
Preventive Services for the Older Adult (65 Years and Older)

    E. Immunizations

• Bivalent diphtheria-tetanus booster	Every ten years
• Pneumococcal immunization	Once only
• Influenza immunization	Initally and annually

    F. Counselling

- Nutrition
- Exercise
- Smoking
- Drugs and alcohol
- Accident prevention
- Self-examination of the breast (women only)
- Self-examination of the genitalia (men only)
- Retirement

From: Modified from Breslow L, Somers AR: The lifetime health monitoring program: A practical approach to preventive medicine. New England Journal of Medicine, 1977;296:601-608.

THE METHODS OF CLINICAL PREVENTION 57

Appendix 3.4
Health Risk Appraisal Program for Mrs. M

DATE: 01-01-1980

YOUR HEALTH RISK DATA HAVE BEEN ANALYZED AND THE RESULTS ARE SUMMARIZED BELOW AS THEY RELATE TO THE 12 MOST FREQUENT CAUSES OF DEATH FOR WHITE FEMALES AGED: 44

RANK	CAUSE OF DEATH	CHANCES OF DYING PER 100,000 WITHIN THE NEXT 10 YEARS			
		COL.1 AVERAGE	COL.2 APPRAISAL	COL.3 ACHIEVABLE	COL.2-COL.3 DIFFERENCES
1	Heart attack	494	887	190	696
2	Breast cancer	464	928	464	464
3	Lung cancer	248	496	397	99
4	Stroke	211	174	68	105
5	Cirrhosis of the liver	190	380	190	¡90
6	Cancer of the ovary	136	136	136	0
7	Suicide	134	268	134	134
8	Intestinal cancer	131	106	32	74
9	Motor vehicle accidents	91	246	52	193
10	Non-Motor vehicle accidents	73	73	73	0
11	Cancer of the cervix	69	69	28	41
12	Diabetes	62	36	33	3
	All other causes	1335	1335	1335	0
	All causes of death	3638	5134	3133	2001

	ACTUAL	APPRAISED	ACHIEVABLE	DIFFERENCE
AGE:	44	48.1	42.3	5.8

For height 67 inches and medium frame 146 LBS. is approximately 4% overweight - - - desirable weight is 140 LBS.

*********************************COMPLIANCE*****************************

Average chances of dying are based on 1975 - 1977 U.S. mortality data. (CDC Version 2.0)

Appraised age (or 'Health Age') is an estimate of how healthy you are compared to others of your race and sex.

Achievable age is an estimate of how healthy you could be by making the following changes in your condition /lifestyle:

Exercise	From:	Undesirable	To:	Sedentary exer. pgm
Smoking	From:	Still smokes 20+	To:	Stopped smoking
Alcohol	From:	7-24/week	To:	3-6/week
Fh/Brest	From:	Family history	To:	Fh + self exam
Papsmear	From:	More than 3 yrs	To:	As recommended
Weight	From:	146 Lbs.	To:	140 Lbs.
Druguse	From:	Sometimes	To:	Rarely or never
Seatbelt	From:	Less than 10%	To:	75 - 100%
Rectexam	From:	No annual exam	To:	Annual exam after 40
S-scale	From:	Above average risk	To:	Risk reduction pgm

NOTE -- Suicide risk is partly based on answers to questions about physical health, life satisfaction, social ties, hours of sleep, recent loss or misfortune and marital status.

Appendix 3.4 (Cont'd.)
Health Risk Appraisal Program for Mrs. M

*** DETAIL *** DATE:01-01-1980

CAUSE OF DEATH	CONDITION	APPRAISAL AS APPRAISED	PARTIAL RISK	TOTAL RISK	ACHIEVABLE ACHIEVED	PARTIAL RISK	TOTAL RISK
Heart attack	Bl. Press	136/86	0.7/0.7		136/86	0.7/0.7	
	Cholestr	Below 220	0.5		Below 220	0.5	
	Diabetes	Not diabetic	0.9		Not diabetic	0.9	
	Weight	146	0.9		140	0.9	
	Exercise	Undesirable	1.4		Sedentary exer. pgm	1.0	
	Smoking	Still smokes 20+	2.1		Stopped smoking	1.1	
	Fh/Heart	No	1.0	1.79	No	1.0	0.39
Breast cancer	Fh/Brest	Family history	2.0	2.00	Fh + self exam	1.0	1.00
Lung cancer	Smoking	Still smokes 20+	2.0	2.00	Stopped smoking	1.6	1.60
Stroke	Bl. Press	136/86	0.7/0.7		136/86	0.7/0.7	
	Cholestr	Below 220	0.5		Below 220	0.	
	Diabetes	Not diabetic	0.9		Not diabetic	0.9	
	Smoking	Still smokes 20+	1.5	0.82	Stopped smoking	1.0	0.32
Cirrhosis of the liver	Alcohol	7-24/week	2.0	2.00	3-6/week	1.0	1.00
Suicide	S-Scale	Above average risk	2.0		Risk reduction pgm	1.0	
	Alcohol	7-24/week	1.0	2.00	3-6/week	1.0	1.00
Intestinal cancer	Rect - Gro	Has not had	0.9		Has not had	0.9	
	Rectexam	No annual exam	1.0		Annual exam after 40	0.3	
	Rect - bld	No blood in stool	0.9	0.81	No blood in stool	0.9	0.24
Motor vehicle accidents	Alcohol	7-24/week	2.0		3-6/week	1.0	
	Miles/Yr	8000	0.8		8000	0.8	
	Seatbelt	Less than 10%	1.1		75-100%	0.8	
	Drug use	Sometimes	1.8	2.70	Rarely or never	0.9	0.58
Cancer of the cervix	Papsmear	More than 3 Yrs.	1.0	1.00	As recommended	0.4	0.40
Diabetes	Weight	146	0.6		140	0.6	
	Fh/diab	No	0.9	0.58	No	0.9	0.54

*************** END ****************

* Risk factors adapted from "How To Practice Prospective Medicine" Drs. Robbins and Hall, Methodist Hospital of Indiana.
* Computer program developed by the center for health promotion and education, Centers for Disease Control, DHHS. (V2.0)
* Adapted for the IBM PC by the Department of Peventive Medicine and Epidemiology University Hospital, Boston MA

NOTE: Health risk appraisal is still in its early stages of development. Its main value is its potential for showing the relative health risks associated with the lifestyle of a particular individual. Since it is a developmental program, it should be interpreted by a qualified health professional.

CHAPTER 4

Preventive Initiatives for Children and Adolescents

Patricia A. Woodbury, C.R.N., M.S.N., C.P.N.A.

INTRODUCTION

Ambulatory pediatrics has come of age and been given the recognition that it has long deserved as a major preventive health care practice. It is now viewed as an integral part of general pediatrics and is in the mainstream of pediatric education. Primary care is only one of the many academic subdivisions of a pediatric curriculum. Many of the "others" also include and are concerned with primary care, eg, psycho-social or behavioral pediatrics, child development, care of children with handicaps, adolescent medicine, child welfare (child abuse and foster care), community pediatrics, school health, and emergency care.

The emphasis of the practice of pediatrics has changed from illness to an interest in prevention and optimal health. For years preventive services were separated from the treatment services, eg, the well-baby clinics versus the physician's office or hospital outpatient clinic where sick care was administered.

Today 33% of visits to pediatric practices are for acute respiratory illness, only 3-10% are for chronic illness, leaving more than half of the child care visits for the well population.[1] Emphasis on prevention is justified, particularly when you consider the years of expected life of the child, as distinct from the adult.

Conceptually, among professional disciplines, the preventive health terminology differs, but within its varied usages there are similarities and agreement. In pediatrics, primary preventive health care encompasses health promotion activities (periodic assessment, anticipatory guidance, developmental counselling), health protection activities (immunization), and prevention of illness services. Screening is the major initiative in the primary level of prevention. Secondary prevention involves early diagnosis of illness and stopping the pathologic process which frequently, in pediatrics, is combined with the services of primary prevention.

This chapter focuses on the first level of preventive health care from the perinatal period through adolescence. The approach and goals of primary prevention will be discussed and compared to those of adult health care.

The chapter presents some of the many preventive initiatives utilized in the delivery of primary prevention to children and their families. Several strategies will be explained in detail.

GOALS AND APPROACHES TO PRIMARY PREVENTION

The desired outcomes for child health are age-related and include: reduction of infant mortality, fostering of optimal childhood development, and improvement in the health habits of youth. Achievement of these goals is dependent, in part, on the constant adaptation of the health care approach to the rapidly developing child, on related health concerns, and on identified risk factors. A discussion follows of some of these goals and approaches utilized in the health care of children.

Adapt the Approach to the Developmental Stage

Primary prevention for children is approached developmentally. Children have significantly different characteristics at different ages or stages in their life; therefore, they are confronted with different health problems and vulnerabilities. For this reason, primary health care must incorporate different approaches to each age or stage. Basically no single packages of care are suitable to all children. Even though the guidelines for health supervision in Table 4.1 are written with specific ages for visits and type of preventive initiative in mind, they are meant to be modified to the unique needs of every child. Different developmental ages in the child have more to do with determining services for health promotion then do disease conditions or chronological age.

Utilize a Broader Approach to Prevention

Today, unlike in the past, childhood mortality from acute disease is rare. Instead, we find chronic and disabling conditions associated with factors other than pathophysiology. The primary health care provider of today must take a broader focus on education of the child, family, and community regarding the multiple causes of illness and disability, eg, housing, nutrition, environment, heredity, stress, and health habits. Chamberlin[2] recommends an "ecologic model" approach to health care. This model focuses on the family and community and the resources therein that can strengthen the functioning of the family unit, as well as improve community mental health.[2]

Part of the process of providing preventive health care is to determine the diseases and impairments you want to prevent for a given population. The child health care provider needs to know not only about pediatric diseases but also adult diseases. Frequently, the poor health conditions in later life have their origins in childhood. As Margaret Heckler[3] has stated, "We are living in a time of unprecedented longevity. To a large extent good health habits determine the quality of

Table 4.1
Guidelines for Supervision of Pediatric Health--Four Stages

Each child and family is unique; therefore these **Guidelines for Health Supervision of Children and Youth**[1] are designed for the care of children who are receiving competent parenting, have no manifestations of any important health problems, and are growing and developing in satisfactory fashion. **Additional visits may become necessary** if circumstances suggest variations from normal. These guidelines represent a consensus by the Committee on Practice and Ambulatory Medicine, in consultation with the membership of the American Academy of Pediatrics through the Chapter Chairmen.

The Committee emphasizes the great importance of **continuity of care** in comprehensive health supervision[2] and the need to avoid **fragmentation of care**[3].

A **prenatal visit** by the parents for anticipatory guidance and pertinent medical history is strongly recommended.

Health supervision should begin with medical care of the newborn in the hospital.

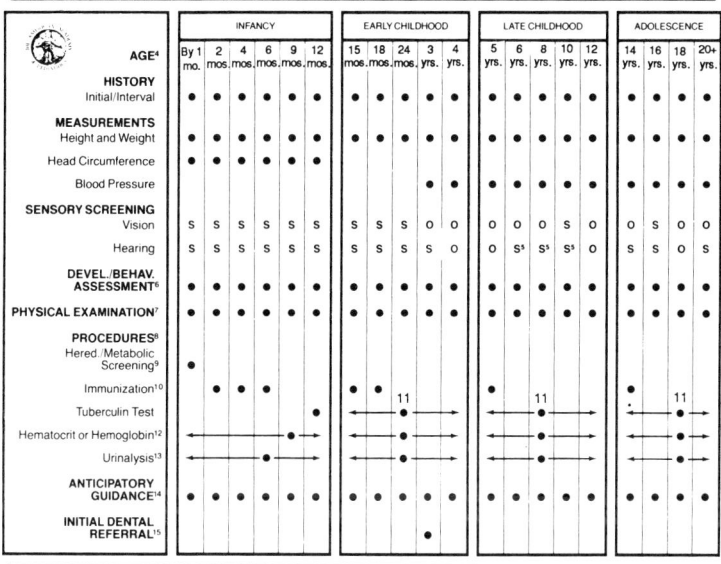

1. Committee on Practice and Ambulatory Medicine, 1981.
2. Statement on Continuity of Pediatric Care, Committee on Standards of Child Health Care, 1978.
3. Statement on Fragmentation of Pediatric Care, Committee on Standards of Child Health Care, 1978.
4. If a child comes under care for the first time at any point on the Schedule, or if any items are not accomplished at the suggested age, the Schedule should be brought up to date at the earliest possible time.
5. At these points: history may suffice; if problem suggested, a standard testing method should be employed.
6. By history and appropriate physical examination; if suspicious, by specific objective developmental testing.
7. At each visit, a complete physical examination is essential, with infant totally unclothed, older child undressed and suitably draped.
8. These may be modified, depending upon entry point into schedule and individual need.
9. PKU and thyroid testing should be done at about 2 wks. Infants initially screened before 24 hours of age should be rescreened.
10. Schedule(s) per Report of Committee on Infectious Disease, ed. 18, 1982.
11. The Committee on Infectious Diseases recommends tuberculin testing at 12 months of age and every 1-2 years thereafter. In some areas, tuberculosis is of exceedingly low occurrence and the physician may elect not to retest routinely or to use longer intervals.
12. Present medical evidence suggests the need for reevaluation of the frequency and timing of hemoglobin or hematocrit tests. One determination is therefore suggested during each time period. Performance of additional tests is left to the individual practice experience.
13. Present medical evidence suggests the need for reevaluation of the frequency and timing of urinalyses. One determination is therefore suggested during each time period. Performance of additional tests is left to the individual practice experience.
14. Appropriate discussion and counselling should be an integral part of each visit for care.
15. Subsequent examinations as prescribed by dentist.

N.B.: **Special chemical, immunologic, and endocrine testing** are usually carried out upon specific indications. Testing other than newborn (e.g., inborn errors of metabolism, sickle disease, lead) are discretionary with the physician.

Key: ● = to be performed; **S** = subjective, by history; **O** = objective, by a standard testing method.

From: News and Comment, May 1982; 33-5. Reprinted by permission from American Academy of Pediatrics.

life in later years." The establishment of good health habits in childhood, eg, nutritious diet, regular exercise, and avoidance of risk-taking behaviors may prevent major health problems such as heart disease, cancer, and stroke in adulthood. Certainly the more positive, health-promoting behaviors the child establishes, the fewer negative behaviors will have to be changed when the child becomes an adult.

In adults, unlike children, the preventive health goals have to be short term, as many potential options for prevention have diminished impact with the passage of time. However, in children the preventive goals are long term and the benefits are not so immediately apparent to the child or his parents. The rewards of these initiatives are delayed, thus frequently decreasing motivation and making compliance less successful. Although parents say they value good health for their children, their own health behaviors are often not productive to these ends. Further it is difficult for the child health care provider to promote these long-term goals when there is no guarantee of the rewards, as many of the preventive initiatives are not yet established. We need to develop short-term goals for children in which some measurable benefits can be experienced.

Maximize the Dynamic Growth and Development of Children

As children are in the stage of active physical growth and development, they have an innate tendency to "self-correct" or "catch-up" following certain disease conditions. Frequently in health care, we feel a compulsion to treat when presented with such conditions or symptoms as bowlegs, fever, or failure to thrive, when in time, these conditions may become more definitive or be resolved. The point here is not to revert to the old adage, "he will grow out of it," but rather to give recognition to the individual child's own pattern and rate of growth and to recognize the limits of preventive health care.

Provide Comprehensive Health Care

Unfortunately, due to cultural factors, a child may still be presented to the health care system with an "acceptable" physical problem when the difficulty may more likely be psychological or family oriented. Currently this trend is changing as child health care providers become more knowledgeable of other health needs and provide counselling for these health problems, be they behavioral or psychosocial. Counseling, to be effective, requires an assessment and understanding of the total family situation and life style. Parenting needs to be rewarded. It is the child health care provider who should provide attention and recognition to parents through honest praise, which will enhance their self-esteem. This strategy may go a long way in the ultimate care of the child and the success in preventive health care.

Establish Mutually Agreed Upon Health Goals

The health professional goals for optimum well-being may not coincide with the child/family or community's health goals. The professional must understand the beliefs and attitudes about health of the family and then develop a "contract" with them that corresponds to their values and life style.

For example, a contract or mutually agreed upon plan of care can be as simple as prescribing an antibiotic for a child with an ear infection. The care giver must impress on the parent the importance of completing the full course of medication. At the same time, the care giver must understand the associated environmental factors that influence the success of the plan. If the child's parents both work, and the child is in a day care center, prescribing a twice a day antibiotic instead of one given four times a day will facilitate compliance with the medical regimen.

A more complex contract is one with an obese adolescent female who would like to lose weight. An understanding of this youth's family life style, and level of development is essential for an effective plan of care. If both parents are obese and not interested in weight reduction, the adolescent will experience difficulty (and stress) in ignoring the parental model as well as their influential eating habits. The status of her self-esteem must be assessed in order to determine the inner strength available to support this young person's expressed goal. Identifying available support systems and resources, eg, school personnel, friends, and community groups, would be important to a proposed weight reduction plan. Simply handing out a specified caloric diet form will be as discouraging as ignoring the overall needs of this adolescent. An informative interchange between the health professional and the patient/family regarding the status of health, recommendations for treatment, and the family's values and resources is imperative for achievement of health goals.

Foster the Child's Independence and Participation in Health Care

Perception of control over health behavior is increasingly recognized as an important determinant of health outcomes.[4] Children need to be educated to take more responsibility for their own health and to learn to use health services appropriately. Children as young as six and eight years are capable of initiating their own visits to a primary care giver such as the school nurse. Each visit to a preventive health care service should be an opportunity for a child, as well as the parent, to develop attitudes of self-help, to diminish dependency, and to participate in his/her own health care.

Provide a Model of Positive Health Habits

Modeling the behavior in others who have successfully achieved the desired goal, can be an effective preventive strategy. Children are great mimics and can frequently be seen modeling the behavior of adults and especially their parents. The "do as I say, not as I do" model has never worked for children nor been effective for other learners. The use of peer models with children has been most effective in such cases of chemical dependency, handicapping conditions, and chronic illness.

For example, Tony, age 12, is a newly diagnosed diabetic. He tells his friend, Mark, that he cannot play on the little league baseball team because he has diabetes. Mark, who is also on the team, surprises Tony by admitting that he, too, is a diabetic. Through the help of his friend, Tony learns to control his diabetes by managing his insulin intake and his diet, so as to fully participate in his favorite sport. Mark provided the model, but Tony recognized that by following the rules of his diabetic regimen he could achieve his desired goal of playing baseball.

In addition to a good model, the child or adult must perceive some incentive or reward for imitating the modeled behavior. While working with adolescent females who wore braces as a nonsurgical treatment of idiopathic scoliosis I had the opportunity to use as a peer model a patient who had a successful therapeutic experience with the brace. Since the peer provided an example of a long-term reward for compliance only, the patient needed some reinforcement on a continual short-term basis. Rewards for compliance, appropriate for a female teen, included periodic purchase of a new dress or blouse after faithful wearing of the brace. Additionally, opportunities to participate in a desired sport, such as swimming, without the brace was also provided as a reward. Positive incentives, perceived as valuable by the patient need to be included in the therapeutic regimen to encourage and support compliance.

PREVENTIVE INITIATIVES IN PRIMARY CARE

Activities occurring at each primary preventive health visit fall under the categories of health promotion, health protection, and prevention of illness. The activities within these categories are routine as well as specific, depending on the age or stage of the child's development.

Health Promotion

Health promotion is a major function of ambulatory pediatrics. The term itself is appropriately descriptive of the services rendered to a relatively well population. These services are aimed at maintaining or raising the quality of life through development of the child's/parent's resources as well as the child's/parent's concious choice or desire for an optimum level of wellness.

Assessment is the first activity of health promotion. This activity includes history-taking and physical/developmental appraisals to create a database of the child/family/community as well as to determine the presence of potential risk factors. The format or content of history-taking varies with each health care provider. The ability to carry out a productive assessment involves interpersonal communication skills along with the knowledge of the health factors associated with this age group.

Table 4.2 is a model of a suggested format for a health promotion visit. This model utilizes a psychosocial developmental approach to data gathering, other than the traditional model. Child health care providers have learned that determining parental concerns in an open-ended, non-directive interview yields more informative data than asking routine, disease-oriented questions.

In assessment of children, the history along with clinical observations frequently provides more information than the physical examination. The results of the physical examination may be affected by the condition or discomfort of the child; and, very often the examiner cannot elicit the reported intermittent signs. For example, a child who has now become tired and irritable after being detained for a long period in the waiting room may not be cooperative in all aspects of the physical examination. A reported intermittent wandering of one eye, by the parent, is sufficient data for referral even though the care giver cannot elicit the symptom during the examination.

If the health care provider maintains an open and accepting approach to data gathering by giving the child or parent permission to talk about their concerns, it is more likely that the attitudes and beliefs held by the family will be revealed, which will affect their health behavior and ultimately the health care plan.

From a preventive perspective, a database should be established as early as possible in a child's life. The child care provider's earliest opportunity is in the third trimester of fetal development when a prenatal visit is encouraged. Under the best circumstances, the mother will have been receiving health care for her pregnancy since the first trimester. Perinatologists believe that prevention of high-risk births is possible through high quality prenatal care. Low birth weight is said to be the most important risk factor in infant mortality. The Institute of Medicine recently concluded that prenatal care is most effective in reducing the chance of low birth weight among high risk women, whether the risk derives from medical factors, sociodemographic factors, or both.[5]

The common prenatal (before birth), intrapartal (during labor), and neonatal (from birth to 28 weeks) complications associated with the birth of a high-risk infant can be divided into two general categories: biologic and psychosocial. The biologic risk factors include: maternal chronic disease, drug addiction, malnutrition, placental abnormalities, neonatal asphyxia, dysmaturity, congenital anomalies, and metabolic disturbances, to name just a few. The psychosocial risk factors include: adolescent parenting, parental psychiatric problems, multi-stressed parent, single parenting, and low socioeconomic status. Most high-risk infants experience more than one risk factor. For example, a premature infant may have an unwed adolescent mother or a woman may

Table 4.2
Health Promotion Visits for Infants--Suggested Formats

2 MONTH VISIT	4 MONTH VISIT
A. Interview 1. How are you? How are things going? 2. Have there been any problems or concerns? Excessive crying? Sleep? Unpredictability of schedule? Unresponsiveness? 3. How is your husband? The other children? 4. What do you and your husband enjoy most about _____? What do you find most difficult about _____'s care? 5. What changes have you seen in development? Social smile? Cooing verbalizations? 6. Return to work? Child care? 7. Any unusual or unexpected family stresses/crises? B. Physical/Developmental/Affective Assessment 1. Plot weight, length, and head circumference. Share with parents. 2. Physical exam with particular attention to strabismus, heart, abdomen, and hips. 3. Parent-infant mutuality and attachment: Cuddling, comforting, verbal communication, infant's responsiveness. 4. Infant's temperament: Fussy, irritable, complacent, passive, actively engaging. 5. Developmental assessment: Direct regard of people; retains objects in hand briefly; social smile; beginning vowel sounds (ah, eh); raises head recurrently when prone; holds head erect when held upright; stops crying when spoken to. C. Immunizations: counsel regarding purpose, contraindications, common side effects; DPT #1, OPV #1. D. Anticipatory Guidance: 1. Nutrition: Stress adequacy of breast and/or formula feedings only, until 4-6 months of age; expectation of more consistent feeding schedule with increasing intervals, expecially at night; "spitting-up" common. 2. Accident prevention: Car safety restraint; rolling off elevated surfaces; toys should be soft, washable without removable parts or sharp edges and large enough not to fit into mouth. 3. Sleep: Schedule becoming established; may sleep uninterrupted for a 12-hour span or awaken every 3-4 hours; stress sleeping in own room and bed. 4. Development: Discuss expected accomplishments over next 2 months; toy suggestions include soft toys that make music, rattles to place in hand, mobile. 5. Other: Ask parents to consult pediatrician regarding use of any proprietary medications; encourage parents to find competent babysitter so they might have an evening out. E. Closing the Visit: Other questions? Compliment. Set return appointment.	A. Interview 1. How are you? How are things going? 2. What problems/concerns have you had since your last visit? Night crying? Resistance when put down to sleep? Crying on separation? Worry about spoiling? Sibling rivalry? Thumb sucking? 3. How is your husband? 4. Have you been out with your husband? 5. What are some of _____'s new achievements? Reaching and feeling with open hand? Laughing out loud? Hand play, mutual fingering? Vocal-social response? 6. Any unusual or unexpected family stresses/crises? B. Physical/Developmental/Affective Assessment 1. Plot weight, length, head circumference. Share with family. 2. Physical exam. Check for strabismus. 3. Observe parent-infant interaction. Evidence of reciprocal vocal and social responses. 4. Observe infant's temperament. Best if defined by parents through interview. Parent's perceptions should regularly be positive even if infant is trying at times. 5. Developmental assessment: Sitting with support; steady head control when upright; rolls prone to supine; hands open at rest; grasps objects near head; takes objects to mouth; several consistent noncrying sounds. C. Immunizations: Again review benefits and risks. Ask about any previous reaction. DPT #2, OPV #2. D. Anticipatory Guidance 1. Nutrition: Stress adequacy of breast and/or bottle. For parents who are adamant about starting solids, rice cereal mixed with formula and fed by small spoon can be added to 1-2 feedings each day. Infant should have a predictable schedule of 4-5 feedings per day. 2. Accident prevention: With increasing motor skills, prevention becomes more important. Playpen convenient and usually accepted at this age; gates for stairways; begin accident-proofing house, i.e., poisons and small objects that might be swallowed. Review management of choking. 3. Sleep. Part-time predictable schedule. Stress own bed and room. 4. Development: Discuss stranger awareness. Encourage play alone in playpen as well as with parents and siblings. Toys to suggest include rattles, spoons, cups, plastic containers and lids, ball to clutch. All should be too large to be placed entirely in infant's mouth. 5. Other: Teething. E. Closing the Visit: Other questions? Compliment. Set return appointment.

From: Green M, Haggerty RJ: Ambulatory Pediatrics III. Philadelphia, PA: WB Saunders Co., 1984. Reprinted by permission develop complications during her pregnancy because she lacked money to obtain adequate prenatal care. Practitioners working with high-risk infants need to understand and be alert to biologic risk factors as well as psychosocial risk factors.[6]

The healthy progress of a child is influenced by the family and the social/emotional/cognitive/physical environment. The social environment includes the nurturing adults and type of emotional climate that is provided to the child. The cognitive environment includes the quantity and quality of stimulation that is provided, especially in the language area. The physical environment is the extent to which a child is provided with sensory learning opportunities as well as predictable, hazard free surroundings.

At times the environment shows indications of disorganization and instability. In those cases, a systematic data gathering initiative must be used to evaluate the child's environment. The Home Observation for Measurement of the Environment (HOME) inventory was designed to sample certain aspects of the quantity and quality of social, emotional, and cognitive support available to a young child within the home. However, administering the HOME inventory is costly and time consuming. An alternative is the Home Screening Questionnaire (HSQ), and adaptation of the HOME inventory. The HSQ consists of two age-appropriate forms (birth to three years and three to six years) that can be completed by parents in the health care office or clinic. The questions in this instrument require a yes/no answer, a check mark beside a listed item, or a short answer. The topic areas cover types of toys and books available at home, location of play materials, opportunities for outside trips, amount and type of play interaction and communication between parent and child. The HSQ is not only quick and economical to administer but accurate in identifying a majority of children whose home environments are substandard (as defined by low scores on the HOME inventory).[7]

Assessing the parameters of growth through measurement of height (length), weight, and head circumference has long been a standard intervention in the health promotion visit. Accurately obtained and plotted physical measurements on standardized growth grids provides a means of identifying possible deviance as well as an educational tool for parents. Figure 4.1 demonstrates the importance of serial measurements. The child's graph might indicate a growth failure, particularly if there was only a single current measure of height and weight. As the pattern of measurements is consistently maintained in the same relative position, however, it most likely suggests a constitutional or genetic factor. It would be important to determine the parental stature as well as the growth parameters of other members of the family.

The National Center of Health Statistics (NCHS) Growth Charts are considered appropriate for assessing the growth of infants, children, and youths in the United States. These percentile curves are based on a large, nationally representative sample of children and reflect a broad consensus of experts in physical growth, pediatrics, and clinical nutrition.[8]

68 HANDBOOK OF CLINICAL PREVENTION

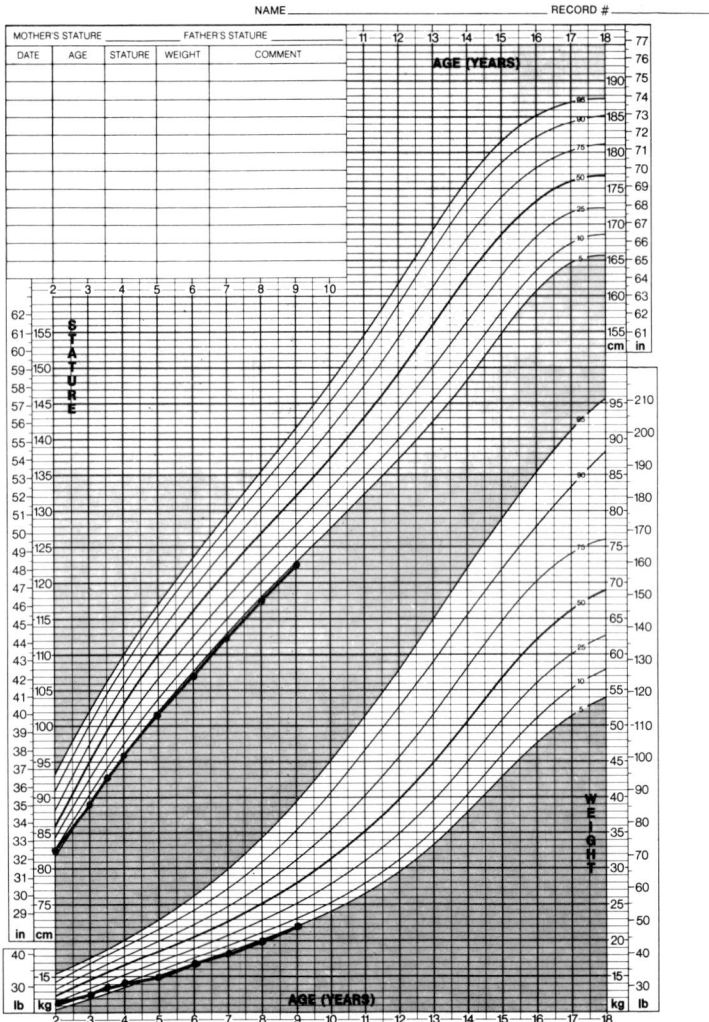

From: National Center for Health Statistics: NCHS Growth Charts. Monthly Vital Statistics Report, 1976;25(3):Supp (HRA) 76-1160. Rockville, MD: Health Resources Administration, June 1976. Data from the National Center for Health Statistics. © Ross Laboratories, Columbus, OH, 1976. Reprinted by permission.

Figure 4.1. Physical growth percentiles for boys 2-13 years: data points represent hypothetical growth pattern of a male patient.

PREVENTIVE INITIATIVES FOR CHILDREN AND ADOLESCENTS   69

The selection of an appropriate developmental appraisal tool requires a decision concerning the desired data. At times the provider may want a tool that determines the level at which the patient is currently functioning in comparison to other children of the same age. At other times the provider may want to identify potential risks to the child. One example of an indirect assessment tool that attempts to identify factors which may lead a child to be at risk for optimum development is the Brazelton Neonatal Behavioral Scale (BNBAS).[9] This scale, developed by T. Berry Brazelton, focuses on the behavior of the neonate towards the environment and to changes in the environment. Figure 4.2 shows a scoring sheet used in this tool. This scale shows that the newborn's capability to control responses to external stimuli within his own environment is varied and complex. Repeated assessments up to one month of age, are of more value than just one assessment completed in approximately 20-30 minutes. There has been no attempt to create a scale whose summary score can be interpreted as "optimal neonatal behavior," since for each baby optimal behavior may be represented by an entirely different cluster of scores. Studies have shown that the BNBAS is a sensitive instrument for predicting developmental outcomes in the neonatal period and for discriminating between abnormal and suspect infants. In addition, this tool is a valuable resource and guideline for teaching parents about their newborn's temperament and individual behavioral patterns. With this understanding parents can be helped to interact appropriately with their own baby.

As the infant progresses and is seen in the ambulatory health care system, other instruments are utilized to observe subsequent development. The Denver Developmental Screening Test (DDST)[10] is the most widely used standardized developmental screening test for children from birth to six years of age. As a first line strategy, it has become useful in the early identification of children with possible developmental delays. The four areas of development assessed in the DDST are personal-social, fine motor-adaptive, gross motor, and language. For each behavior an age range is given that indicates when 25%, 50%, 75% and 90% of the children perform the task. The DDST is not an IQ test but merely a tool for determining where a child is, in comparison with his peers, in the performance of certain tasks. A child with a questionable or failing score should be referred for further testing. The DDST is a valuable developmental teaching tool for parents, as well as a tool for identifying children at risk.

The major tasks of the school age-child surrounds learning. Frequently, the primary health care provider is requested to contribute to the assessment of a potential learning problem in this age child. Appraisal of any child with school failure involves a systematic, comprehensive approach including historical review, physical, neuro-developmental, and psychological assessments. This assessment process demands the interdisciplinary cooperation of many health and school professionals. The primary care provider's contribution is the basic health history, physical, and neurodevelopmental information. These findings should assist in the determination of the need for further neurological or specialized consultation.

Behavioral and Neurological Assessment Scale

Infant's name		Date	Hour
Sex	Age	Born	
Mother's age	Father's age	Father's S.E.S.	
Examiner(s)		Apparent race	
Conditions of examination:		Place of examination	
Birthweight		Date of examination	
Time examined		Length	
Time last fed		Head circ.	
Type of delivery		Type of feeding	
Length of labor		Apgar	
Type, amount and timing of medication given mother		Birth order	
		Anesthesia?	
		Abnormalities of labor	

Initial state: observe 2 minutes

1	2	3	4	5	6
deep	light	drowsy	alert	active	crying

Predominant states (mark two)

1	2	3	4	5	6

Elicited Responses

	O*	L	M	H	A†
Plantar grasp		1	2	3	
Hand grasp		1	2	3	
Ankle clonus		1	2	3	
Babinski		1	2	3	
Standing		1	2	3	
Automatic walking		1	2	3	
Placing		1	2	3	
Incurvation		1	2	3	
Crawling		1	2	3	
Glabella		1	2	3	
Tonic deviation of head and eyes		1	2	3	
Nystagmus		1	2	3	
Tonic neck reflex		1	2	3	
Moro		1	2	3	
Rooting (intensity)		1	2	3	
Sucking (intensity)		1	2	3	
Passive movement		1	2	3	
Arms R		1	2	3	
L		1	2	3	
Legs R		1	2	3	
L		1	2	3	

Descriptive paragraph (optional)

Attractive	0	1	2	3
Interfering variables	0	1	2	3
Need for stimulation	0	1	2	3

What activity does he use to quiet self?
hand to mouth
sucking with nothing in mouth
locking onto visual or auditory stimuli
postural changes
state change for no observable reason

COMMENTS:

O* = response not elicited (omitted)
A† = asymmetry

From: Brazelton TB: Neonatal Behavioral Assessment Scale (2nd edition). Philadelphia, PA: JB Lippencott, 1984. Appendix 1, pp. 114-115. Reproduced with permission by MacKeith Press, London, England.

Figure 4.2. Brazelton neonatal behavioral assessment scale.

Behavior Scoring Sheet

Initial state
Predominant state

Scale (Note State)	1	2	3	4	5	6	7	8	9
1. Response decrement to light (1,2)									
2. Response decrement to rattle (1,2)									
3. Response decrement to bell (1,2)									
4. Response decrement to tactile stimulation of foot (1,2)									
5. Orientation—inanimate visual (4,5)									
6. Orientation—inanimate auditory (4,5)									
7. Orientation—inanimate visual and auditory (4,5)									
8. Orientation—animate visual (4,5)									
9. Orientation—animate auditory (4,5)									
10. Orientation—animate visual and auditory (4,5)									
11. Alertness (4 only)									
12. General tonus (4,5)									
13. Motor maturity (4,5)									
14. Pull-to-sit (4,5)									
15. Cuddliness (4,5)									
16. Defensive movements (3,4,5)									
17. Consolability (6 to 5,4,3,2)									
18. Peak of excitement (all states)									
19. Rapidity of build-up (from 1,2 to 6)									
20. Irritability (all awake states)									
21. Activity (3,4,5)									
22. Tremulousness (all states)									
23. Startle (3,4,5,6)									
24. Lability of skin color (from 1 to 6)									
25. Lability of states (all states)									
26. Self-quieting activity (6,5 to 4,3,2,1)									
27. Hand-to-mouth facility (all states)									
28. Smiles (all states)									
29. Alert responsiveness (4 only)									
30. Cost of attention (3,4,5)									
31. Examiner persistence (all states)									
32. General irritability (5,6)									
33. Robustness and endurance (all states)									
34. Regulatory capacity (all states)									
35. State regulation (all states)									
36. Balance of motor tone (all states)									
37. Reinforcement value of infant's behavior (all states)									

From: Brazelton TB: Neonatal Behavioral Assessment Scale (2nd edition). Philadelphia, PA: JB Lippencott, 1984. Appendix 1, pp. 114-115. Reproduced with permission by MacKeith Press, London, England.

Figure 4.2 (Cont'd.). Brazelton neonatal behavioral assessment scale.

The Neurodevelopmental Screening Examination[11] was developed at Children's Hospital Medical Center in Boston by Melvin Levine, MD and associates. It is an age-normed test that assesses the aspects of developmental competence, minor neurological signs, gross motor ability, fine motor function, visual processing, sequential organization and memory, and language competence. This pediatric neurodevelopmental battery's major contribution to the multidisciplinary evaluation process is in the form of a descriptive versus a psychometric model. That is, the tool in combination with other data and input from other disciplines, becomes a narrative description of a child's strengths and deficits rather than an overall numerical score which might be misleading. In addition, the neurodevelopmental screening tool can reveal to the patient, parents, and care provider, insights regarding the child's attention patterns, functional styles, and coping mechanisms. These assessment initiatives provide the basis by which the focus of the next educational intervention is determined.

Health education takes many forms depending on the setting, number of persons involved, chronological age of the patient, stage of development, or presenting concern on the part of the patient and/or provider. In the pediatric primary care setting, health education is provided in the form of anticipatory guidance. Anticipatory guidance is a preventive health tool that the primary care giver uses to structure health teaching. The structure is age-dependent, and the content is those physical and behavioral changes that parents can generally expect in their child. The object is to prepare parents in advance for normal childhood developmental changes, thereby increasing their understanding and enjoyment of their parenting role.

Anticipatory guidance is probably most unique to pediatrics because of the child health care provider's focus on development as well as this age population's dynamic stage of life. The content areas are the known sequence of events that every child experiences. For example, anticipatory guidance routinely includes developmentally oriented information about nutrition, feeding behaviors, accident prevention, developmental states, sleep behavior, elimination training, and discipline. Traditionally, anticipatory guidance is provided on a one-to-one basis between provider and patient/parent, at the time of the periodic assessment visit.

Another format for anticipatory guidance is group education. Prenatal classes for the expectant parents have been offered, most usually by obstetrical staff of a hospital. Through these classes, parents are guided through the process of fetal development, birth, and neonatal care. In addition, they learn how to foster good health habits for the benefit of both mother and child. This preventive initiative helps to avoid maternal/parental stress during pregnancy, labor, and delivery. Frequently following birth, many parents continue with a parent group which is organized to build support and provide information that enhances the competence and confidence of first-time parents.

The curriculum, presented by a trained facilitator, contains a wide range of topics matched to the parents' immediate needs, as well as the anticipated topics of health, child development, family management, or personal development. More specifically, these groups of parents discuss how to select a primary care provider; what information to bring to a preventive health visit; how to arrange more time for baby, spouse, and self; and how to become wise consumers of baby products. These parent groups may be organized within a community education program or within the primary health care setting itself.

Another form of education that has developed in recent years within the community is early childhood parent education programs. These programs are supported by legislated revenue that is distributed through local school districts. They serve children from birth to kindergarten and their parents. By providing quality programs that teach parents how to educate and interact with their children, the child is given a head start. Potential learning problems are identified, and families learn that they are a vital part of their child's education and learning.

By school-age, the child is a direct recipient of health education. The setting for this education may be in a formal class or it may be a "teachable moment" when a student comes into the health office for first aid or illness.[12] Today many school systems are providing more than a one-time talk on health by means of an ongoing formal health curriculum required from kindergarten through 12th grade. The curriculum links health information with interactive programs to promote life style change. A variety of subjects are taken up including physical fitness, accident prevention, alcohol and drug use, sex education, dental health, personal hygiene, stress reduction, crisis intervention, and use of health resources.

Implicit in health education is the concern with prevention of illness as well as an emphasis on influencing individual behavior. A program that exemplifies this approach is called Know Your Body (KYB).[13] This is a school health education system which combines screening of selected risk factors, a personal health passport of screening results, a behaviorally oriented curriculum, and specific high risk interventions. The screening techniques include measurements of blood pressure, blood cholesterol, height/weight/skinfold thickness, and physical fitness--as determined by pulse rate recovery after a stepping up and down exercise. The curriculum is divided into two levels, elementary and junior high school. The overall objectives of the curriculum focus on increasing health knowledge, reinforcing positive feelings about ones body, promoting personal responsiblity for health, encouraging change in health practices to reduce health risks, and promoting healthy life style practices. Success with this program requires the support and participation of the medical community, teachers, and parents.

Some drawbacks to this program were cited by both Walter and Connelly.[14] The cost of this screening program was found to be substantial in terms of equipment, laboratory costs, and personnel. Walter expressed concern regarding accuracy and inferences drawn from screening results. For example, the high rate of false positive blood pressure measurements were considered outside of normal. There was also a concern for increased anxiety from labeling participants as "abnormal." To avoid this, results were presented as either "optimal" or "less than optimal." Participation by students was high for the non-invasive procedures such as, growth measurements, but low for more threatening procedures such as the blood and fitness tests.

When dealing with older children a mutual understanding of the purpose and type of test being provided is imperative to achieve favorable outcomes for the program. Also, protection of individuals, rights, including confidentiality, must also be stipulated in health education programs for young people.

On the positive side, the KYB program can elevate health education to the level of other major curriculum areas in the schools. The program increases the students' awareness of the relation of a physical parameter to health and disease. The teacher's role, both as an educator and a participant in the program incorporates the general principles of social learning theory, including modeling, behavioral rehearsal, goal specification, feedback, and reinforcement for positive behavior change.

Another form of health education in the school has been the "Health Fair." Multiple health stations providing information about specific health risks, eg, hypertension, nutrition, stress, and fitness, are set up in the school. Many community health organizations contribute to the success of these fairs. This is an opportunity for students to meet various health representatives from their community, and ask questions about their own health risks and fitness. Through these various educational modes, the school-age child is learning about self-care.

Self-care is an approach to health care that makes the patient, rather than the health provider, the primary health source. It is the self-initiated and self-controlled application of knowledge that is necessary for the promotion of health.[15] In 1976, John Knowles,[16] then President of the Rockefeller Foundation, wrote: "The next major advances in the health of the American people will result from the assumption of individual responsibility for one's own health." Health professionals who are adverse to this concept fear that the provider-patient relationship will be jeopardized and that the patient will avoid using the health facility on the basis of less than sound clinical judgements. The proponents of the concept believe that self-care encourages more positive health behaviors. By taking a more active role in their own self-care, patients are learning what to do in an emergency, eg, first aid, CPR, prevention of injuries and self-maintenance of health records, and prevention of infections of the respiratory or urinary systems.

Project Health PACT (Participatory and Assertive Consumer Training) is one example of a program for school-aged children which teaches them how to participate with health professionals in making decisions about their health and health care.[17] Childhood is the best time to foster an

PREVENTIVE INITIATIVES FOR CHILDREN AND ADOLESCENTS   75

assertive health consumer role, rather than the traditional adult passive health consumer role. Active problem-solving behavior on the part of the child and/or consumer is key to health promotion, protection, and disease prevention.

Health Protection

Health protection refers to action that focuses on controlling environmental factors such as immunization, fluoridation of water, and sanitation. These are a few of the legislated health protection measures. The responsibility for these measures are outside the individual's control and benefit the general population.

Identification of environmental hazards should be integrated into the pediatric health care provider's assessment of each child-patient and family. Table 4.3 provides a developmental guideline to some of the potential environmental hazards that may compromise a child's health. Exposure to hazardous chemicals and radiation are especially problematic during fetal development. Such chronic disorders as retardation, minimal brain damage, and altered immunologic response in very young children have been linked to exposure to noxious substances. Frequently, the subsequent problems related to a child's exposure to hazardous substances are not evident for many years. Exposure to pesticides in food, water, or atmosphere is a problem that extends from fetal life throughout childhood. Unlike adults, children are more vulnerable to these chemicals because of the proportionally low body weight per exposure. Lead poisoning in children has been a well known hazard for years, associated with brain damage, poor school performance, and slow development.[18]

Immunization is a mainstay of preventive initiatives in health protection. Immunization prevents the occurrence of an infectious disease by introducing an antigen or antibody that will confer protection without making the person unduly sick. Vigorous efforts on the part of private and public health care delivery systems to immunize the population at risk have had a dramatic impact on the control of infectious diseases in our country. Since 1978, most states have passed legislation for compulsory immunization regulations. The schedule for active immunization for normal infants and children recommended by the American Academy of Pediatrics is shown in Table 4.4. Education of parents is a must for increased compliance with immunization schedules. Parents need specific information about each vaccine including nature, prevalence, risk of infection or disease, nature of the product used, expected benefits of the vaccine, possible or likely side effects, risk of rare but serious adverse effects, role of the vaccine in developing immunity, and any needed followup to complete the immunization. Explaining how the child's immunization is related to the entire community's health, may enhance motivation to complete the vaccine schedule.

Table 4.3
Assessment of Risk
Environmental Exposure: Children and Youth Matrix

CATEGORY	PRENATAL (fetus)	INFANT	CHILD	YOUTH
Chemical substance	Cigarette smoking ··			
	Drugs ··· Ingestions (household toxins/prescriptions) ······ Drug use (street and OTC)			
	Mercury (teething powders/ anthelmintics ·············			
	Pesticides, insecticides ······· Asbestos (parental occupational dust) ··········· Occupational hazards			
	Airborne pollution ·············			
	Toxic waste ····			
		Formaldehyde (Insulation) ·······································		
Ionizing radiation	X-ray pelvimetry	Skull x-ray (overuse)	Dental x-ray (overuse)	
Heat and fire	Fumes from gas and woodburning stove	Flammable fabrics	Hot stoves, matches	Heat illness
Electricity		Exposed wall sockets, cords and wiring ·········		
Kinetic energy		Infant seats (misuse)		
		Car seats (lack of use) ·····		
		Stairway gates (lack of) ···		
			Jungle gyms	
			Bicycles, skate boards ········	
			Sports injuries ·············	
		Transportation injuries ···		
Infectious agents	Viral/bacterial/microbial infections ···			
		Animal/insect bites ···		
Air and water quality	Airborne pollution ···			
	Ozone - smog ···			
		Contaminated drinking water ··		
		Unfluoridated water ····································		
		Drowning ··············		
Social stress		Physical abuse ···		
		Unsafe toys ············		
			Firearms ···································	
		Violent crime ···		

····· indicates continued exposure

Table 4.4
Recommended Schedule for Active Immunization of Normal Infants and Children

SERIES	AGE	PREPARATIONS	REFERENCE
PRIMARY	2 months	DTP - TOPV	1, 2
	4 months	DTP - TOPV	
	6 months	DTP - TOPV	3
	12 months	Tuberculin test	4
	15 months	Measles, mumps, rubella	5
	24 months	*Haemophilus influenzae,* type b	7
BOOSTERS	18 months	DTP - TOPV	
	4-6 years	DTP - TOPV Tuberculin test	6
	14-16 years	Td, repeat every 10 years Tuberculin test	

Abbreviations: DTP : Diphtheria, tetanus, pertussis vaccine
Td : Tetanus, diphtheria (adult) vaccine
TOPV: Trivalent oral polio vaccine
Hib : *Haemophilus influenzae,* type b

1. This recommendation is suitable for breast-fed as well as non breast-fed infants. DTP and TOPV may be started as early as six weeks. Intervals between doses of DTP and TOPV may be as close as six weeks.

2. Trivalent Oral Poliovirus Vaccine (TOPV) is not recommended for infants with immune deficiency disease or receiving immunosuppressive therapy.

3. This third dose of primary series TOPV is optional in the United States. It should not be given unless there is a history of vomiting and diarrhea suggestive of viral gastroenteritis occurring five to seven days after polio immunization. The reason for administering this dose should be documented on the immunization record.

4. If the inital tuberculin test is not given at 12 months of age, it may be given at the time of the measles-mumps-rubella (M-M-R) immunization. Do not delay the M-M-R immunization by waiting for the tuberculin test to be read. All tuberculin tests should be done with 5TU intradermal (Mantoux) test.

Table 4.4 (Cont'd.)
Recommended Schedule for Active Immunization of Normal Infants and Children

5. Although optimum antibody response is obtained when M-M-R immunization is deferred until 15 months of age, if a child who is at least 13 months of age is presented for immunization, the child should be immunized for measles, mumps and rubella unless absolute assurance can be obtained that the child will return for immunization at 15 months of age.

6. Persons six years of age or older should not receive pertussis (Whooping Cough) vaccine. If six years of age or older, Td (Adult) vaccine is recommended. DT (Pediatric) may be substituted for those under six years of age who have had reactions to DTP.

7. Haemophilus influenzae type b vaccine has not been shown to be effective in children under 18 months old. The primary dose should be given at age 24 months or between the ages of two and five years if previously not immunized. It is also recommended for children age 18 to 23 months who have sickle cell anemia, asplenia or are in other groups at high risk for Haemophilus influenzae type b infection, including children in day care centers.

Accident prevention: In recent years, child health care providers have become more involved with other health protection strategies directed toward the prevention of childhood accidents. In the past, society's attitude toward accidental death and injury has been fatalistic. The belief was that accidents were "bad luck" and beyond human control. A more recent view, however, is to identify the factors involved in accidents and apply preventive interventions.

The three main factors involved in accidents are: the individual, the agent, and the environment. For example, the curious, ambulatory toddler (individual), toxic cleaning fluids, if ingested (agent); and an unlocked cupboard in an unsupervised kitchen (environment) together make for a potential accident. Similarly, a young, inexperienced bike rider in dark clothing (individual and agent), on a dark, rainy night, riding on a loose, gravel shoulder, on a road with heavy traffic (environment) creates another accident situation. These are only two of many incidences of potential injury in which children may find themselves. By recognizing the individual developmental characteristics of the child as they relate to the environment and associated agent, educational efforts may be developed to prevent accidents in anticipated circumstances.

Automobile safety is an especially important area of accident prevention. Automobile related accidents are the number one cause of death in children. Sixty percent of these deaths or injuries can be prevented by proper use of child auto restraints. During the last five years, 49 states have enacted child passenger safety laws. Child health care providers must direct injury prevention efforts toward those who possess the power to affect the environment in which children live. This target group most likely would be the child's parents and/or family. However, it seems that the governmental regulatory agencies have a greater impact on preserving the health of our children given the statutes for car seats, day care, toxic agent control, and child abuse reporting.

Protective activities for school-age children include many of the preschool topics for safety. Because of the increasing physical skills and risk-taking behaviors of this age group, safety programs need to include additional topics including bicycle safety; swimming survival skill; protective sports equipment; driver education; sex education, including contraception and sexually transmitted disease; and substance abuse education. Health education efforts for youth should present positive alternatives to risk-taking behaviors rather than just pointing out the pitfalls of these behaviors.[18]

Teenage pregnancy prevention. Unprotected sexual activity is a major risk-taking behavior among youth today. Ten percent of females, aged 13 years, and 14% aged 15 acknowledge having had intercourse. The percentage increases to 46% by 19 years of age.[19] The Guttmacher Institute[20] found that many teenagers experiment with sex for months before ever using contraceptives. As a result, about 62% of these sexually active teenagers experienced a premarital pregnancy compared to 30% of those who used a contraceptive method, although inconsistently.

Teenage pregnancy in the United States, according to a 1985 Guttmacher Institute Study, is virtually epidemic, surpassing other nations of the Western world.[21] The main difference in the United States, compared to other nations, is our attitude toward sex. A powerful message is delivered through the media by means of advertisement. For example, ads for underwear, designer jeans and deodorants often include explicit sexual content. Unfortunately, very little is included either about the risks involved in sexual activity, such as pregnancy and sexually transmitted disease, nor that youth have an alternative choice to sexual activity.

Most pregnancy prevention programs thus far have been in the form of secondary prevention. We have provided pregnancy testing, prenatal clinics, and child day care. Contraceptive education and access has only been offered after an initial pregnancy. Preventing adolescent pregnancy involves intervention on a number of levels. The goal of primary prevention here is to prevent the initial pregnancy.

In public schools where classes do exist, most sex education is limited in content and scope, addressing only the basic issues of anatomy and physiology of human reproduction. There is an increasing effort to change the focus of sex education to include the developmental issues surrounding the etiology of sexual behavior among youth. For example, some adolescents' lack of ability to plan ahead, as well as their "it can't happen to me" thinking, makes it less likely that they will use contraceptives. Equally important is the understanding of the factors that contribute to active sexual behavior, such as the need for love, desire to get even with parents, adventure, ignorance, the need to validate masculinity or femininity, the need to maintain peer popularity and acceptance, and the need to counter insecurity and fear.[22] These are the aspects of sexuality that adolescents need to understand and discuss through educational programs, for it is only when sex is viewed as a deliberate action that the teenager can begin to accept responsibility for such behavior and make informed choices.

In the last decade, preventive initiatives toward reduction of teenage pregnancy have shown evidence of success. The St. Paul Maternal-Infant Care (MIC) project has served as a model for clinics situated in the high school setting. Their measure of success, as with other school-based clinics, is lower fertility rates, improved contraceptive continuation rate, fewer high school students lost to followup, and increased number who graduate from high school.[23,24] Factors contributing to these measures of success included: easier access and availability of student and staff; consistent, confidential, and free services; inclusion of both teenage partners; special focus on the youth's perception of needs, concerns, and fears.[24]

Dryfoos[23] puts on a par access to reproductive health care with access to education and employment. He feels that the core of preventive strategies is in the creation of a "life option;" that is, to provide young people with a stronger rationale for avoiding pregnancy through broadened horizons, elevated self-esteem, and activities emphasizing career options.

Prevention of Illness

The final category of primary prevention is the early identification of disease and the prevention of illness and disability. An exemplary strategy of this point is immunization which is considered health promotion, health protection, and prevention of illness. A basic difference between disease prevention and health promotion is that health promotion strategies focus on wellness and the strategies of disease prevention are directed toward a specific illness.

Screening is the major initiative of illness prevention. Screening can be used for early identification of disease, both before a disease is present as well as in a subclinical stage of disease. Tables 4.5 and 4.6 present the many preventive health and screening procedures utilized in the care of children from birth through adolescence.

Screening is the application of a quick, simple, and accurate test to an asymptomatic population to separate those who have a problem from those who do not. Several conditions should be present before screening begins.
- The potential problem must be important—either of fairly high frequency (visual problems) or great severity even if infrequent (hypothyroidism).
- There must be agreed-upon criteria for diagnosis of the condition.
- The potential problem being assessed must be more effectively treated in the asymptomatic phase, and effective treatment must be available.

The screening test itself must have sensitivity (ability to detect all who have the problem), specificity (ability to test only those with the problem), and predictive positives. If false positives are too high, the cost of referral and followup make the test less useful.

Table 4.5
Age Specific Screening Procedures: Package for Newborns

CONDITION/DISEASE	TEST(S)	TREATMENT IN RESPONSE TO POSITIVE TEST(S)
Birth defect/disease/ maternal illness	APGAR score Gestational age	Intensive care, monitoring
Phenylketonuria	Test of phenylketones in the urine	Diet therapy
Neurological	Neonatal Behavioral Assessment Scale (Brazelton)**	Parent counseling and follow-up
Hypothyroidism* (cretinism)	Serum thyroxin	Appropriate thyroid hormone replacement therapy
Emotional maldevelopment	Neonatal Perceptual Inventory (Broussard)†	Counseling for parenting skills
Galactosemia	Galactose in blood	Galactose free diet
Atherosclerosis	Serum total cholesterol (cord blood)	Appropriate diet
Erythroblastosis fetalis	Coombs' test, hemoglobin, bilirubin (cord blood)	Exchange transfusion Phototherapy for increased bilirubin
Congenital hip dysplasia	Ortolani test	Orthopedist referral

* This should be prevented by adequate iodine in the diet of the mother.

** Brazelton TB: The Neonatal Behavioral Assessment Scale. Philadelphia: J.B. Lippincott, 1973.

† Powell ML: Assessment of Maternal Perceptions of Infants. Assessment and Management of Developmental Changes and Problems in Children, second edition. St. Louis: C.V. Mosby, 1981.

Table 4.6
Age Specific Preventive Health and Screening Procedures: Children and Youth Packages.

CONDITION/DISEASES	TESTS(S)	2 WKS	1 2 4 6 9 12 15 18 MONTHS	3 5 8 11 14 16 18 YEARS	TREATMENT IN RESPONSE TO POSITIVE TEST(S)
Marasmus & obesity	Weight Triceps skinfold thickness Length and OFC Height	• •	• •	• • • • • • • • • • • • • • • • • • • • •	Diet counseling
Iron deficiency anemia	Hematocrit or hemoglobin		• • • •	• • • • • • •	Iron therapy
Lead poisoning	Free erythrocyte protoporphyrin (FEP)		• • • •	•	Drug therapy
Poor vision	History or risk factors Response to light/ alignment/reflexes Snellen chart	• •	• • • • • • • • • • • • • • • •	• • • • • • • • • • • • • •	Referral to opthamologist
Delayed hearing/ speech development	History of risk factors Reaction to sound, vocalization Pure tone screen	• •	• • • • • • • • • • • • • • •	 • • • • • • •	Referral to hearing or speech pathologist
Sickle cell trait	Sickle cell prep		•		Additional testing
Congenital dislocation of hip	Physical examination	•	• • • •		Appropriate orthopedic referral
Primary hypertension	Family history Blood pressure measurement (sphygmomanometer)	•	• • • • • • • •	• • • • • • • • • • • • • •	Nutritional counseling and other appropriate hygienic measures Drug stepped care
Tuberculosis	PPD skin testing (pre-MMR and annually/biennially depending on local circumstances) (chest film for previously known positive tuberculin test)		•	• • • • • • chest x-ray	Isoniazid or other appropriate chemo/ antibiotic therapy

Table 4.6 (Cont'd.)
Age Specific Preventive Health and Screening Procedures: Children and Youth Packages.

CONDITION/DISEASES	TESTS(S)	AGE 2 WKS / 1 2 4 6 9 12 15 18 MONTHS / 3 5 8 11 14 16 18 YEARS	TREATMENT IN RESPONSE TO POSITIVE TEST(S)
Urinary tract infection	Quantitative urine culture	MONTHS: • (15) ; YEARS: • • • • • • •	Chemo/antibiotic therapy
Skin disorders (acne)	Skin assessment	2 WKS: • ; MONTHS: • • • • • • • • ; YEARS: • • • • • • •	Referral or appropriate therapy, including anti-acne treatment regimen
Dental problems	Oral/dental screen	2 WKS: • ; MONTHS: • • • • • • • • ; YEARS: • • • • • • •	Referral to dentist
Diphtheria/pertussis mumps/rubella	Immunization documentation	MONTHS: • • • (2,4,6) • (18) ; YEARS: • • (adult Td)	Thereafter Td every ten years
Polio/measles mumps/rubella	Immunization documentation	MONTHS: • • • (2,4,6) • (15)	
Health risks (abuse, eating disorders, pregnancy, suicide)	Interview for: safety, environmental factors, drugs, nutrition, accidents, sex, etc.	2 WKS: • ; MONTHS: • • • • • • • • ; YEARS: • • • • • • •	Educate for safety, environmental, factors, drugs, nutrition, accidents, sex Appropriate referral
Developmental abnormalities	Denver Developmental screening Test (DDST)	MONTHS: • • • • • • • • ; YEARS: • •	Monitor or refer for further evaluation
Scoliosis	Structural clinical signs, forward bend	YEARS: • • • • •	Refer for spine x-ray and orthopedic consultation
Precocious or delayed puberty	Physical examination Tanner's Staging	YEARS: • • • • •	Monitor or refer to endocrinologist
Sexually transmitted diseases	Smear/culture	YEARS: • • •	Appropriate drug therapy
Testicular cancer	Testicular examination	YEARS: • • •	Appropriate referral

In children, hearing and vision problems are present in only one in every 100 children. However, developmental problems are present in as many as one in five children. Developmental assessment was discussed earlier in this chapter. The American Academy of Pediatrics suggests that every child have a test of visual acuity by four years of age. Most visual defects are errors of refraction. Approximately 5% of first graders have such problems, but almost 50% of children develop them by the end of high school. Strabismus (cross-eyed) and anisometropia (inequality of the focus of the light rays on the retina of both eyes) are present in 1-5% of school-aged children.[25] The Snellen[26] test identifies most children with vision problems. Young children may be better tested with the E form of the Snellen test or by Sheridan's Test for Young Children and Retardates (STYCAR)[27]. The child is asked to focus on a distant object while one eye is covered. If the child has esotropia (deviation of one eye inward) or exotropia (deviation of one eye outward), when the cover is removed, the eye that has wandered will immediately resume its straight-ahead position.

The American Academy of Pediatrics recommends that every child have a hearing test by four years of age. Pure tone audiometry is the test of choice. In audiometry, the ear is exposed to a series of pure tones of calibrated loudness (decibels) occurring at different frequencies ranging from 250 to 6000 Hertz (Hz). Approximately 5% of elementary school-aged children do not pass hearing screening tests. Upon retesting, several weeks later, about half of those previously failing will pass. This pattern is probably the result of upper respiratory infections, fluid in the middle ear, misunderstood instructions, or lack of attention.

Two preventive initiatives or self-screening techniques that have long-term implications are breast examination and testicular examination. Teenage females should be instructed in the procedure of breast self-examination (BSE). Although most masses discovered during adolescence will be benign, the long term value of this initiative is in the establishing of a good health habit, as well as baseline data for later reference. Similarly, the adolescent male should be instructed in the self-examination of the scrotum. Malignant testicular tumors have a peak incidence in late adolescence and early adulthood. Early detection can reduce the serious and potentially fatal consequences of malignancy.[28] Another value of teaching testicular self-examination (TSE) early is the establishement of a good health habit and an understanding of normalcy.

<u>Early Identification of Risk Factors: Example Coronary Artery Disease.</u> Many of the risk factors in coronary heart disease have been shown to have their roots in infancy and childhood. These include hyperlipidemia (an excess of fat or lipids in the blood, obesity, and hypertension. The current recommended nutritional guidance for the young infant includes preventive initiatives relative to coronary artery disease. Mothers who prefer to breastfeed their baby are encouraged to do so for the first six months of life. All mothers are cautioned about introducing solid foods before four months of age. Parents receive advice concerning prepared infant foods and the avoidance of additional salt and sugar in the diet.

Families in which the children are at high risk for developing obesity, due to the presence of one or more obese family members, deserve special attention. Attention is indicated also for those children at high risk for cardiovascular disease as identified by family history. A program of preventive health care should be implemented for high risk children. The content for this program should be individualized according to the following assessed areas:

- family life style regarding attitudes toward, and role of, food;
- eating patterns and associated stimuli;
- snacking (including types of food and frequency); and,
- the importance of physical activity and exercise in everyday life.

There is a significant relationship between obesity and hyperlipidemia. Screening of children with a family history of coronary heart disease is recommended for evidence of elevated serum cholesterol (a waxy substance with fat-like properties found in blood, muscle, brain, liver, and all human/animal cells) or triglycerides (major transport and storage form of fatty acids). Children with elevated cholesterol values (greater than the 95th percentile) at two successive examinations, two years apart, are reported to have a two-fold increased risk of coronary mortality.[29] Preventive initiatives for these children would include a diet low in cholesterol and high in polyunstaturated fat. For the infant, this would indicate breast milk or use of a proprietary formula. For the older child, reduction of red meat in the diet along with the use of 2% milk would be advisable.

The reported incidence of hypertension in the pediatric population varies from 0.6-11%. The variability in prevalence rates is directly related to age and the criteria used to define hypertension.[30] Currently, an elevated blood pressure must be present in at least three separate examinations over a six- to 12 month interval, if not associated with other signs or symptoms. Figure 4.3 and Figure 4.4 provide the procedure for identification of asymptomatic children and the normogram for plotting the measurements.

For those patients with sustained blood pressure levels, treatment may include either weight reduction, dietary sodium reduction or pharmacologic management, or all three. In addition physical activity appears to be helpful in the amelioration of obesity, hyperlipidemia, and hypertension.

The effects of exercise training on known coronary risk factors have been found to be valuable in altering these factors in adults. It is postulated that exercise will have a similar effect on children. Although there is not sufficient longitudinal data available on child/adolescent exercise, regular physical activity during childhood may serve a two-fold purpose. It will minimize the development of coronary disease during adulthood and set a pattern for a physically active life throughout childhood and adulthood.[29] Compliance with an exercise program is more

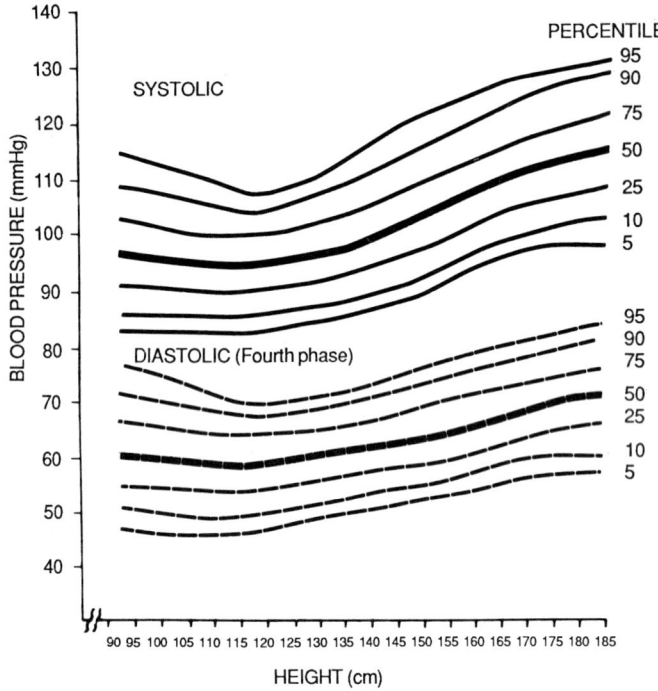

From: Berenson GS, Cresanta JL and Webber LS: High blood pressure in the young. Annual Review of Medicine, 1984;35:536-559.

Figure 4.3. Percentiles of blood pressure measurement for boys.

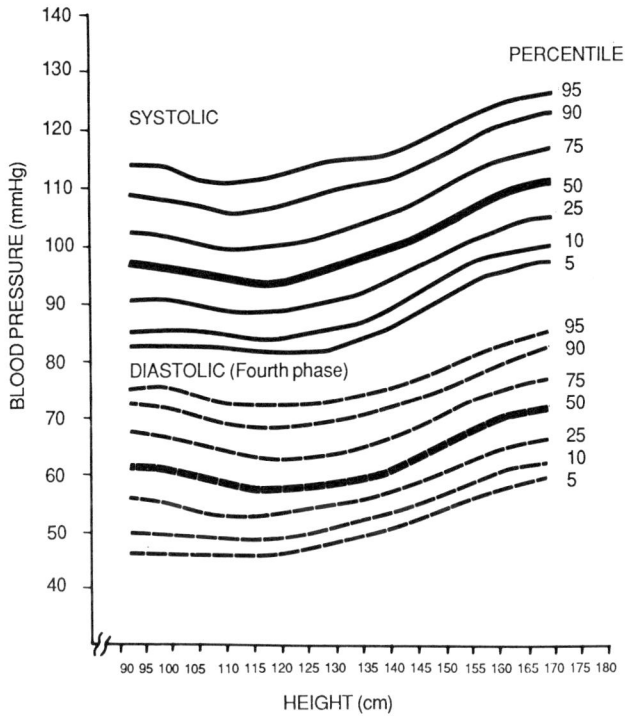

From: Berenson GS, Cresanta JL and Webber LS: High blood pressure in the young. Annual Review of Medicine, 1984;35:536-559.

Figure 4.3 (Cont'd). Percentiles of blood pressure measurement for girls.

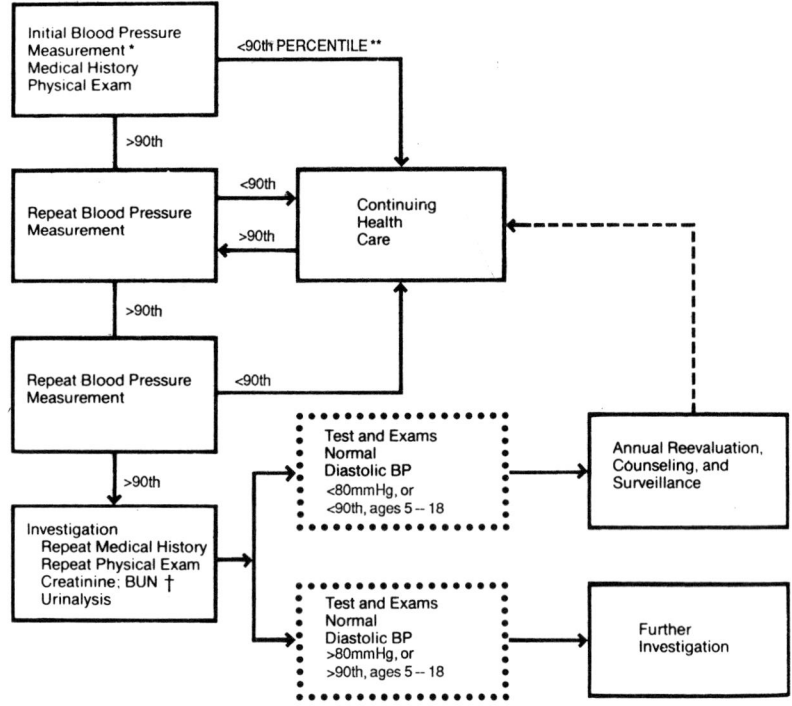

Blood pressure measurements should be made at 1-4 week intervals.

* If initial blood pressure measurement taken at school or other community center, two subsequent blood pressure measurements should be made prior to referral of patient, if feasible.

** The 90th percentile is an arbitrary statistical cutoff point; children with blood pressure at the 90th percentile should be labeled as having high normal pressure rather than being hypertensive.

† Optional: If patient is obese or a cause identified for hypertension, BUN or creatine may not be indicated.

From: Algorithm adapted from The Task Force on Blood Pressure in Children: Standards for children's blood pressure. Pediatrics, May 1977 (supplement);59:802-803. Reproduced by permission of Pediatrics.

Figure 4.4. Identification and evaluation of asymptomatic children with elevated blood pressure.

likely if it is individualized in consideration of the patient's interest, capability, and physical status. The health care provider who serves as a role model through personal participation in regular exercise will help to encourage such activity in the patient.

Unfortunately, health education of the consumer has been more affected by the manufacturers of children's toys, cereal companies, and producers of television programs than by health professional initiatives. The marketing of health promotion information is a major challenge for today's health care professionals. Child health care providers in particular must become more visible in the media, community education programs, public service clubs, school lectures, health advisory boards, and legislative efforts where health information is needed and health policy is being formulated. Child health advocacy has been an integral part of pediatric practice for a long time. Continued application of each of these preventive initiatives (role modeling, consumer awareness, and advocacy) by child health care providers is needed to influence public perception regarding major causes of morbidity and mortality.

SUMMARY

Primary health care for children has been contrasted to primary health care for adults. Selected goals and approaches were cited to show this difference. A few of the many interventions utilized in primary prevention for children were discussed to illustrate the difference as well as the relatedness of child health to adult health.

Due to the generally good health of children, health care efforts are mainly focused on the primary prevention level. Because of the influence of the environment, including family and community, on the health of the child, the pediatric primary care provider must consider, if not work directly with, not only the child-patient but also the parents, other family members, school personnel, day care providers, and potentially other community health resources.

The provider of primary health care of children must have a flexible approach because of this dynamic stage of life. The many preventive initiatives are applied in accordance with the current developmental level of the child.

The future of health care seems to be directed towards a more reciprocal relationship between the highly trained professional and a better educated client. Children need to learn early about self-care, the appropriate use of health care resources, and how to be an active participant in their own health care.

In primary prevention, particularly with children and youth, a positive model is suggested that addresses positive health alternatives and outcomes versus negative consequences. The therapeutic plan will be more acceptable if developed through mutual understanding and agreement of the professional and client. Compliance with the health care plan is more likely when long-term as well as short-term incentives or rewards are included and perceived by the child/ youth-patient.

Health education is perhaps the most powerful intervention in preventive health care. The awareness level of parents and adults in the community about the potential risk factors impinging on the health of children must be raised through use of as many educational formats as possible. Finally the currently best known preventive initiatives should be introduced in order to support a healthy life style and avoid, or at least delay, potential health problems.

REFERENCES

1. Green M, Haggerty RJ: Ambulatory Pediatrics III. Philadelphia: WB Saunders Co., 1984.

2. Chamberlin RW: Strategies for disease prevention and health promotion in maternal and child health: The "ecologic" versus the "high risk" approach. J Public Health Policy 1984:185-195.

3. Heckler MM: Health—Make it last a lifetime. Public Health Reports 1984;99:221-222.

4. Chalmers K, Farrell P: Nursing interventions for health promotion. Nurse Practitioner 1983;8:62-64.

5. Institute of Medicine: Preventing low birthweight. IN: Report of the Committee to Study the Prevention of Low Birthweight. Washington, DC: National Academy Press, 1985.

6. Davis DH: Ongoing nursing care of the high-risk infant. IN: Mott SR, Fazekas NF, James SR (eds.): Nursing Care of Families and Children. Menlo Park, CA: Addison-Wesley Publishing, 1985.

7. Bradley RH: The home environment: Effects on the development of children. IN: Children Are Different: Behavioral Development Monograph Series (number 15). Columbus, OH: Ross Laboratories, 1985.

8. Hamill PVV, Moore WM: Contemporary growth charts: Needs, construction, and application. IN: Public Health Currents. Columbus, OH: Ross Laboratories, 1976.

9. Brazelton TB: Neonatal Behavioral Assessment Scale. No. 88 - Clinics in Developmental Medicine Series. Philadelphia: JB Lippincott Co., 1984.

10. Frankenberg WK et al.: Denver Developmental Screening Test: Reference Manual (revised edition). Denver, CO: LADOCA Project and Publishing Foundation, 1975.

11. Levine MD, Brooks R, Shonkoff JP: A Pediatric Approach to Learning Disorders. New York: John Wiley and Sons, 1980.

12. Wold SJ: School Nursing: A Framework for Practice. St. Louis: C.V. Mosby, 1981.

13. Williams CL: Risk reduction in the schools: The "know your body" program. IN: Faber MM, Reinhardt AM (eds.): Promoting Health Through Risk Reduction. New York: MacMillan Publishing Co., 1982.

14. Walter JH, Connelly PA: Screening for risk factors as a component of a chronic disease prevention program for youth. J School Health 1985;55:183-187.

15. Fletcher DJ: Self-care. Postgrad Med 1985;78:213-223.

16. Roemer MI: The value of medical care for health promotion. Amer J Pub Health 1984;74:243-248.

17. Igoe JB: Project health pact in action. Amer J Nursing 1980;80: 2016-2021.

18. Robinson GC: Prevention of illness. IN: Mott SR, Fazekas NF, James SR (eds.): Nursing Care of Families and Children. Menlo Park, CA: Addison-Wesley Publishing, 1985.

19. Blum RW, Goldhagen J: Teenage pregnancy in perspective. Clin Ped 1981;20:335-340.

20. Alan Guttmacher Institute: Teenage Pregnancy: The Problem That Hasn't Gone Away. New York: Alan Guttmacher Institute, 1981.

21. Yates S: U.S. far exceeds other nations in teen pregnancy. Health Link 1986;2:45-46.

22. Jackson VD, Kidwell JS: Curbing the rising tide of teenage pregnancies in the U.S.: Primary preventive approaches for communities, schools, and parents. Health Values: Achieving High Level Wellness. 1980;4:269-273.

23. Dryfoos JG: A new strategy for preventing unintended teenage childbearing. Family Planning Perspectives 1984;16:193-195.

24. Edwards LE, Steinman ME, Arnold KA, Hakanson EY: Adolescent contraceptive use: Experience in 1,762 teenagers. Amer J Obstes and Gyn 1980;137:583-587.

25. Green M, Haggerty RJ: Ambulatory Pediatrics III. Philadelphia: WB Saunders Co., 1984.

26. Snellen H: Symbol Test of Visual Acuity: Snellen Illiterate E. New York: National Society for Prevention of Blindness, 1970.

27. Sheridan M: STYCAR Vision Test Manual (2nd revised edition). Windsor, Berks, England: NFER Publishing Co., 1970.

28. Williams HA: Screening for testicular cancer. Ped Nurs 1981;7:38-40.

29. Moorehead C, Rocchini AP, Rosenthal A: Risk factors to coronary artery disease and ways to alter them. Pediatric Basics. Gerber Products Co., March 1984; number 37.

30. Weil WB: Obesity in children. Pediatrics in Review 1981;3:180-189.

ADDITIONAL READINGS

Brandt EN: Infant mortality-A progress report. Public Health Reports. May/June 1984;99:284-290.

Brandt EN: Prevention as a policy. Public Health Reports. September/October 1982;97:399-401.

Castiglia PT, Petrini MA: Selecting a developmental screening tool. Ped Nurs 1985;11:8-17.

Krassner L: TIPP usage. Pediatrics (supplement—Patient Education). November 1984;74:976-978.

Lazar I: Lasting Effects After Preschool. U.S. Department of Health, Education and Welfare, Office of Human Development Services. Publication No. 79301790, 1983.

Pender NJ: Health Promotion in Nursing Practice. Norwalk, CT: Appleton-Century-Crofts, 1982.

Robert Wood Johnson Foundation. The perinatal program: What has been learned. Special Report, number 3, 1985.

Strain JE: AAP periodicity guidelines: A framework for educating patients. Pediatrics (supplement—Patient Education). 1984;74:924-927.

Wiebe RA: Ambulatory pediatric care. IN: Kelley VC: Practice of Pediatrics. Volume 1. Philadelphia: Harper and Row Publishers, 1982-1983.

Watkins AC: How about a health fair? Ped Nursing 1983;9:123-126.

CHAPTER 5

Behavior Models and Methods for Preventive Health Programs

Robert C. Benfari, Ph.D.

The last 15 years have seen the birth and growth of behavioral medicine. This philosophy recognizes that the most cost effective approach to the delivery of health care services and prevention of many diseases is to employ behavioral techniques to promote lifestyle changes. Behavioral and environmental interventions have the potential to improve the life expectancies of a great number of individuals. These interventions can improve compliance to medical regimens and, more importantly, alter risk factor behaviors in order to prevent disease. A large body of literature analyzes the effectiveness of various techniques for both compliance and prevention. It is not our purpose to review or to recapitulate these works.[1-3]

This chapter focuses on the application of behavioral intervention techniques to preventive medicine/health care. Past experience with diverse target behaviors and populations has demonstrated that, in spite of the techniques used, roughly one third of the participants change their behavior in the course of the program. The mechanisms for this type of behavioral change are not clearly understood, although multiple hypotheses, including the placebo, pygmalion and Hawthorne effects have been formulated. Participants in behavioral change programs are 'easy riders' who appear to be highly motivated and do not have self-limiting behavioral deficits. Relatively simple and efficient intervention techniques can work for these individuals.

The results of the cigarette cessation component of the MRFIT program illustrate this point.[4,5] Smokers who smoked a pack or less of cigarettes and were motivated to change accounted for 70% of the initial change in the program. On the other hand, the high dose smokers had a significantly lower rate of cessation, in spite of their desire to change. The intervention program was designed to focus on three risk factors using a ten-session group format. These intervention techniques worked well for the low-risk smoker but were not as effective for the high-risk smokers. In terms of effectiveness of preventing coronary heart disease (CHD), the latter group presented the greater need. This chapter is devoted to the problems of high risk individuals, the ones most in need of intervention, who present the greatest challenge to the intervention program. Simple and easy solutions are not usually effective with this target population. In all fairness to the fledgling interventionist, it must be pointed out that there are no clear-cut solutions to these complex cases. Therefore, one must approach the problem of behavior change with a sense of realistic expectations, both positive and negative, about the limits of behavior change. In spite of well intentioned participants and highly motivated interventionists, failures and unexpected successes will always occur. The intent of the chapter is to present a model that deals with the complexities and challenges of behavioral intervention.

THE BEHAVIOR PROBLEMS IN PREVENTIVE HEALTH CARE

Behavior change in preventive medicine presents a different set of problems and considerations than behavioral compliance in curative medicine. In the former instance, the interventionist is usually concerned with altering risk factors rather than curing a set of visible or recognizable symptoms. The latter case usually involves:

- A sickness and possibly some incapacitation
- Some curative process
- The responsibility of a cure in the hands of a trained practitioner

It has been pointed out in many cases that this framework has limitations when the behavior change involves risk factors. Baric[6] has labelled this condition as the "at-risk" role where the following prevail:

- The role is not institutionalized.
- It endures for an indefinite time span.
- It has no continuous reinforcement from the health care system and the social environment.
- It does not provide feedback from changes in symptomology or treatment procedures.[6]

Under these circumstances, the interventionist must utilize motivating mechanisms which differ from those used when the patient is in the sick role. For example, it is necessary to make the participant aware of the following:

- The change is desirable because it will have specific positive consequences;
- The participant can acquire the necessary knowledge and skills to carry out the change;
- The change is in his/her self-interest;
- The change is in the best interests of the family;
- The key to behavior change lies in responsibility assumption;
- The intervention program is designed to develop specific skills in this area.[7]

Using these concepts the intervention takes on a problem-solving approach. For example:

- What are the problem areas of the participant?
- What are the strengths and weaknesses of the participant?
- What environmental factors facilitate or prevent change?
- What consequences does the problem have for the participant and significant others?
- What satisfactions would continue for the participant if the problem behavior were to continue?
- What satisfactions woul occur if the behavior were changed?
- What new problems would develop as a result of behavioral change?
- What adverse effects would develop for others if the behavior change occurred?
- Is the participant capable of undertaking the intervention program?

When this approach is used, a cognitive based behavioral program can be developed.

THE ROLE OF THE INTERVENTIONIST:

Primary Tasks

The key assumptions in our model of behavior change are:

- The interventionist influences the participant by encouraging responsibility assumption.
- The interventionist offers pathways to new behaviors.
- The ultimate decision for behavior change rests with the participant.
- Therefore, only the participant can change his/her behavior.

The assumption of responsibility is the keystone to behavior change. As long as the participant avoids this factor there is no internal commitment to change. The focus of the participant remains external and most likely he will exhibit all of the classical defenses for avoiding awareness of responsibility. In order to achieve the overall objective of responsibility assumption, the interventionist must accept this as an overarching frame of reference. The other alternative is to become the agent of change and run the risk of producing excessive dependency in the participant. This assertion does not imply that the interventionist is passive and not supportive of the participant but rather that the interventionist must always come back to the role that the participant plays in determining his/her life script(s). The ability to assume responsibility, like most behaviors, will be differentially distributed among individuals. More will be said about measuring this propensity in a later section. For the present discussion we will focus on the pitfalls that the interventionist must be aware of in the participant's desire to avoid responsibility. By becoming aware of these pitfalls, the interventionist can prevent the building of a dysfunctional therapeutic alliance. The interventionist's strategies will make the participant aware of these avoidance tactics and turn the problem of behavior change over to the participant.

THE PROBLEM OF RESPONSIBILITY AVOIDANCE

It is a frightening thought that we are mainly responsible for our situation in life. Somehow it is more comforting to think that we are driven by circumstances and events rather than by our own actions or inactions. Since this theme has been given extensive coverage elsewhere, we do not attempt to demonstrate its validity but accept it as an existential fact of life. The role of the interventionist is to facilitate the process of confronting responsibility avoidance and move the participant toward awareness of possibilities and willful decision making. Yalom,[8] in discussing responsibility avoidance, has described five defensive mechanisms that patients/participants will exhibit when they attempt to avoid responsibility assumption. They are:

- compulsivity;
- displacement of responsibility to another;
- denial of responsibility (innocent victim, losing control);
- avoidance or autonomous behavior; and
- decisional pathology.[8]

Compulsivity

Compulsivity is manifested when participants maintain they are controlled by some outside forces that determine their behavior. Some examples of compulsive behavior are binge eating, habitual smoking, workoholism and drug/alcohol dependency. Participants are aware only of the need and perceive the factors at best as ego-alien (not me determined).

Displacement of Responsibility

Patients/participants maintain that someone else is causing the problem. This could be within the family, the work situation, or in social relationships. The focus of the problem is the other person, not themselves. This defense is different from compulsivity in that another person(s) are part of the belief system rather than an irrepressible force.

Denial of Responsibility

INNOCENT VICTIM

The participants avoid responsibility by explaining their behavior as a victim of events that just happen to them. For example: "I was at the party and everyone was smoking, drinking, or eating; and I had to go along with the crowd." Or: "I was at a business lunch and was forced to eat the filet mignon." The participants do not see that they had a choice in the matter but feels victimized by circumstance.

LOSING CONTROL

Whereas participants who perceive themselves as innocent victims have an awareness of the behavior, there are others who cite their unconscious as the cause of the behavior. "I lost control and found myself in the situation." This defense is clearly a desire for nurturance and understanding from the interventionist. The participants portray themselves as the victim of their unconscious desires. Another way of putting this is that "the devil made me do it."

Avoidance of Autonomous Behavior

Even when the participants are aware of what they can do to help themselves, they do not take the necessary steps to correct the situation. This defense points out that awareness by itself is not enough to achieve behavior change. The participant must accept the fact that only they can change the situation through willful action.

Decisional Pathology

The key factor in this defense is the inability of the participants to come to terms with ambivalence toward behavior change. That is to say the participants have contradictory intentions. They want to change their life circumstances but at the same time value the behavior that must be given up. Sometimes this is experienced in a sequential fashion where the participants at one moment vow the need but at another time repudiate the act. Or it can be experienced simultaneously, where the conflict of intentions is directly confronted. The latter arouses considerable anxiety but offers a direct approach to the resolution of the ambivalence. (The interventionist's strategy should be to convert sequential to simultaneous ambivalence so that the ambivalence is experienced in a here-and-now fashion.)

STEPS FOR INTERVENTION

The first step for the interventionist is to beware of the issues and to catalog the events. These events become specific data points for discussion with the participant. When the interventionist is certain that one or more of the avoidance symptoms are present, he or she can focus the participant's attention on the specific instance in the here and now and relate back to similar instances of this behavior. The objective is to make the participant aware of the excuses for non-performance by labeling the behavior. The participant and the interventionist now have a common understanding of the event. The interventionist's role is to ask the participant to "own" the behavior. From this point the interventionist's task is to awaken the participant to the possibility that "cannot" statements are really "will not" statements and that responsibility for any behavior is our own. Some interventionists use the technique of the "can't" bell—where they ring a bell or some similar device to ask the participant to change "cannot" to "will not." This simple technique forces the participant to assume responsibility. The intervention procedure is enhanced in groups whereby the interventionist can use the resources of the group membership to develop awareness of their avoidance of responsibility. Yalom[8] points out that the participant learns about responsibility assumption through the following sequence:

1. Participants learn how their behavior is viewed by others. Through feedback, and later through self-observation, participants learn to see themselves through others' eyes.

2. Participants learn how their behavior makes others feel.

3. Participants learn how their behavior creates the opinions others have of them.

4. Participants learn how their behavior influences their opinion of themselves.

These forms of interactional therapy enhance responsibility assumption. The group leader can focus on here and now examples of responsibility avoidance and use these to focus on individual issues. The group leader may also wish to allow other group members to become adjunct facilitators.

SETTING THE CLIMATE FOR INTERVENTION

In order to move toward participant responsibility assumption, the interventionist should be concerned with the creation of a positive learning environment. One of the critical factors in achieving long-term behavior change is the interventionist-participant interaction. In this regard Chris Argyris[9] has has done some relevant research on the creation of learning environments. Argyris draws upon White's[10] work on motivation, which shows that individuals need a sense of competence in order to become more effective in human interactions. If individuals can be shown alternatives or pathways toward more effective behavior, they will strive to utilize this behavior because it satisfies the need to be competent. This assumption is the bridge between the defenses against responsibility assumption and taking charge of one's life. If we accept competence seeking as the overarching motivator, our job as interventionists is to create the appropriate environment in order for the participant to move in that direction. Argyris has defined two distinct learning environments that have opposite behavioral outcomes.[9] He calls them Model I and Model II Environments. These two learning environments seem to have direct application to the interventionist-participant interaction and their outcomes. For example, Model I consists of four action strategies:

1. One person (interventionist) defines the goals and the way to achieve them.

2. The control of the therapeutic task remains solely with the therapist.

3. Feelings and emotions of the participant are minimized.

4. There is a tendency to withhold information.

In this climate the participant sees the interventionist as inconsistent and controlling, norms are established between the two, and low internal commitment is developed on the part of the participant. The ultimate goal of responsibility assumption is sabotaged by the learning environment. The outcome of a Model I environment is at best short-term compliance and dependent behavior. Kelman[11] describes such behavioral outcomes as compliance and identification which are based on short-term rewards and penalties rather than on internalization and responsibility assumption.

On the other hand, Model II is governed by the following action strategies:

1. The interventionist's role is to generate valid information and to create a situation in which the participant has a sense of high personal involvement in the process (mutual causation).

2. The decisions are based on free and informed consent and the task of change is jointly controlled. The interventionist facilitates adoption of alternatives and pathways. The participant is the decision maker.

3. There is an attempt to achieve internal commitment to the decisions and to explore any pitfalls to achieving competent behavior.

In this climate of interchange, controlling behavior, and defensiveness are minimized since the interventionist acts as a facilitator and the participant develops responsibility assumption and personal causation, and is motivated by competence seeking.

THE ROLE OF EXPECTATIONS IN THE THERAPEUTIC ALLIANCE

Recent research by Luborsky[12] has identified the following three key factors in the development of a positive working arrangement between the interventionist and the participant.

1. The participant believes that the interventionist knows the problem and that he (the participant) is gaining new understanding and hope for future behavior change.
2. The participant trusts the interventionist and his ability to help him.
3. The participant and the interventionist have common expectations. The participant feels that he and the interventionist share common ideas about his problems and about treatment, and is not trying to impose his own views.[12]

The last factor appears to be one area where more effort on the part of the interventionist can be profitably expended. Whether or not expectations are shared, they are part of every human interaction. A psychological contract is formed based upon previous experiences, future expectations with regard to goals, roles, and procedures. If the psychological contract (therapeutic alliance) remains implicit, there is a high potential for conflict. For example, a participant may have the expectation that the interventionist will take responsibility for his behavior or provide excessive support during stressful times. This situation will clearly violate Luborsky's third principle. Another common expectation that needs to be shared and dispelled is "the negative self-fulfilling prophecy." In this case the participant anticipates failure and sets himself up for the negative outcome. Under these circumstances the interventionist's job is to make the participant aware of this belief system and to discuss means for developing competent behavior. On the other hand, the positive self-fulfilling prophecy, based on realistic goals and means of attainment, can be a powerful motivator and subsequent reinforcer (see Table 5.1).

The therapeutic alliance (positive psychological contract) can be strengthened if the participant and interventionist openly discuss the following topics:

- Their perceived goals in the relationship
- Mutually agreed on strategies
- Whether the goals and strategies relate to the central needs of the participant
- A challenge or sense of competence experienced by the participant in meeting his goals

The therapeutic alliance is by nature a dynamic relationship. Needs and expectations change over time. Therefore, even if they are addressed early on, they may have to be revisited at other junctures in the intervention program. If they are not addressed early in the relationship, the interventionist is setting himself up for conflict and most likely failure.

Table 5.1
Problem Expectations

PARTICIPANT EXPECTATIONS	INTERVENTIONIST EXPECTATIONS
Anticipation of failure based on previous experience, low self-esteem, fear of success, or the negative self-fulfilling prophecy	Anticipation of failure based on unacknowledged biases
Expecting psychological dependency in the therapeutic relationship; The interventionist will take care of the problems	Expecting to maintain unilateral control of the intervention process
Expecting magical outcomes; Just by showing up something will happen	Expecting a rational, realistic approach by the participant
Having divergent or incompatible goals to the outcome of the intervention; Expecting something different than outcome will happen	Expecting the participant to share his goals
Expecting simple or easy pathways to change	Acceptance of difficulties
Using the intervention for hidden agendas	Expecting a simple goal oriented approach by the participant
Expecting unqualified support from the interventionist	Expecting the participant to be self-supporting

MEASURING RESPONSIBILITY ASSUMPTION

At the present time no psychometric instrument exists that directly measures responsibility assumption. On the other hand, for the purposes of clinical diagnosis rather than scientific validity, it is possible to come close to assessing responsibility assumption by using the Rotter Internal/External Locus of Control Index.[13] This instrument measures the degree to which individuals feel governed by an internal versus external locus of control. This variable has been correlated with positive outcomes of behavior change in many studies. It has also been demonstrated that externals, when compared to internals, have greater feelings of inadequacy, have more inclination toward hopelessness, are lower in achievement orientation, and are less likely to succeed in stopping smoking. Based on these results, the Internal/External scale offers the interventionist an opportunity to assess the participant's/patient's propensity for avoiding responsibility. The results can be used as feedback to participants to counter this tendency. Under the guidelines of generating valid information and informed consent, it can be a powerful means for both the interventionist and the participant to deal with this aspect of the intervention process. Using shared information, with clear expectations on the part of both parties, enables them to face the problem more expeditiously. In this case assessment instruments are part of the intervention process and are used as a paradigm for behavior change.

The following steps could be part of the intervention program:

- Have the participants take the Rotter Internal/External Index.
- Introduce the concept of responsibility assumption to the participants in a group session devoted to discussing barriers to effective behavior change.
- Have the participants write out scenarios of times when they attempted to change their behavior (the behavior should be related to the one under consideration).
- Share the results of the Rotter with the participants and explain its significance.
- Correlate the results of the Rotter with the scenarios. This step brings the abstract assessment results closer to actual behavior, as recounted in the scenarios.
- Have the participants discuss the personal relevance of the results for their behavior change.

PERCEPTUAL CHANGE: A PARTICIPANT GOAL

Many participants in a preventive health program are unaware of the viable options or choices for decision making. Their perceptions about possible changes are fixated on past experience or even based on erroneous assumptions or beliefs. In the broadest sense, assumptions are based on our past perceptions and experiences, or on the perceptions or observations of others. These assumptions prescribe the way it ought to be and ultimately drive our behavior. Regardless of the therapeutic approach, an alteration in the participant's assumptive and perceptual views may be necessary to provide altered expectations of upcoming situations and potential resources. In addition to altering expectations, some serious barriers to performance may be uncovered during this phase of intervention. For example, some cultural or ethnic groups will have beliefs about the role of certain foods in providing physical and spiritual sustenance. Unless these issues are explored they may become impediments to changing the problem behaviors. One of the more time-honored approaches is called cognitive restructuring and was first documented by Ellis[14] and expanded upon by Lazarus[15]. Ellis contended that the extent to which an individual labels a situation as positive or negative influences emotional responses and behavior patterns. In some instances the perception and self-beliefs may be inaccurate, inappropriate, or irrational.[14]

In order to implement the cognitive restructuring procedure, a four-step approach is taken:

1. Demonstrate to the participants that they are illogical; help them to understand how and why they became so, and demonstrate the relationship of irrational ideas to emotional and behavioral responses.

2. Demonstrate to the participants that they are maintaining those undesired emotions and behaviors by continuing to think illogically—that is, that it is their present irrational thinking that is responsible for their present state, and not the continuing influence of early events.

3. Help the participants change their thinking and abandon the irrational beliefs and self-verbalizations.

4. Develop a more rational philosophy of choices so that the participants are not trapped by past assumptions and perceptions.

Cognitive restructuring approaches have been used for smoking cessation, weight control, stress management, and drug compliance, in addition to more general psychological disturbances as depression, unrealistic goals, and self-defeating behavior. Many psychologists have attempted to vary and objectify the rational-emotive therapy advocated by Ellis. These variations focused on increasing the development of a cognitive restructuring skill, which could then be used as a self-help coping tool for future problem situations. The basic goal in all of these approaches is to have the participant identify internal dialogues related to the problem behavior, evaluate these self-statements for their rationality and influence on behaviors, and then produce new self-statements that are incompatible with the original beliefs and problem behaviors. Goldfried[16] and his colleagues developed the following procedures:

- The client is provided a rationale of the approach.
- The participant is given an overview of some typical irrational assumptions.
- The participant is taught to recognize and modify his/her self-verbalizations that are associated with the undesired behavior through imagination or role play.
- The participant is instructed to assess the level of anxiety/emotional upset experienced during this process as a cue to signal any self-defeating thoughts or statements made during the imagined situation, the role-play situation, and for future situations (i.e., "What am I telling myself that may be irrational?").
- The participant is instructed to reevaluate these self-statements and to replace them with more realistic, appropriate statements, after which another assessment of the anxiety-emotional upset level is made. The participant is told that this procedure is deliberate and tedious at first like the learning of any new skill. With practice, however, one can expect to find each step easier and more natural.

Through this process, the interventionist can help the participants realize that they can cope more effectively with a probabilistic world based on rational choices rather than on undeveloped ruminations.

Behavioral Contracting

Since both the participant and the interventionist enter the therapeutic relationship with their own set of expectations, it is a necessary step in good intervention practice to explore these individual expectations and to develop a shared set of mutual expectations and responsibilities. The process by which this "psychological contract" is derived is called behavioral contracting. The first step in the process is to share expectations about the intervention procedure(s) and outcomes. The second step is to adjudicate any unrealistic or unrelated expectations and to focus on the goals and objectives of the intervention program. These steps help to uncover any hidden agendas on the part of the participant such as expecting major help in social-emotional areas when the main focus is on other target behaviors (smoking, eating habits, weight control, etc.). The third step in behavioral contracting takes place when the participant is expected to modify specific target behaviors. Stuart[17] has isolated the following main elements for an effective contract.

- Specify the desired behaviors and responsibilities of each party involved.
- Specify the rewards or penalties that can be expected with the fulfillment or nonfulfillment of the above stated behaviors and responsibilities.
- Detail a method by which the rewards or penalties will be administered.
- Allow for additional reinforcement for extended periods of appropriate behaviors.
- Include or identify a monitoring system to record the compliance of the terms stated.

THE USE OF PSYCHOLOGICAL TESTING IN BEHAVIOR CHANGE PROGRAMS

In recent years behavioral interventionists have moved toward the use of many standardized psychological tests to help both the interventionist and the participant to understand themselves and, as a result, become more competent and effective in the intervention program. Since the intervention effort is viewed as a transaction between the therapist and the participant, it is necessary that these psychological tests should be used as indicators of strengths and weaknesses in both parties. This use of the psychological tests removes them from the realm of diagnosis or control, only in the hands of the therapist, to a collaborative role. The instruments that could be used include those measuring stress levels, assessing the participant's social environment, and measuring the preference styles of the participant. The latter assessment has some important considerations for the design of specific intervention programs and for the fit between the therapist and the participant. Not everyone perceives, makes judgments, or comes to a decision in the same manner.

At this point we are introducing the variable of individual differences as a factor in the therapist/participant interaction. In another section of this chapter, the role of the therapist/participant interaction was alluded to as important in determining the outcome. At that time some general rules for conducting an intervention program were introduced as guidelines toward generating a more effective intervention climate. Based upon previous research with learning environments and outcomes, it would seem profitable to focus on objective data that could be generated for both the therapist and the participant to understand their preferences in perceiving and judging. The Meyer Briggs Type Indicator (MBTI)[18-20] has undergone extensive psychometric validation by the Educational Testing Service (ETS) and other investigators since the late 1960s and is currently being used in many applied contexts. Examples include use by medical students to help them choose an appropriate specialty, use by teachers to design curriculum for different types of students, use by therapists[20a] to understand their patients, and wide use in organizational development. The theory behind the MBTI is based upon Jung's model of psychological functions. An extensive knowledge of psychological theory is not necessary, however, to use the MBTI and its concepts in an applied setting. In addition, the concepts are neutral and nonpejorative in meaning. They phenomenologically differentiate people on four dimensions (Figure 5.1). The concept of preference is similar to handedness. Although we have two hands, we develop a preference of one over the other.

1. Extraversion (E) vs. Introversion (I): This dimension measures how persons will use their psychological energy. Extraverts find energy in things and people in the world outside of themselves. They are pulled by this outer life of action and spend less time with inner thoughts and concepts. Introverts find energy in their inner life of ideas, concepts, and abstractions. They have a rich inner life and therefore seem to require less of the outside world. In the general population of the United States, the prevalence of extraversion (E) to introversion (I) is 75% to 25%.

2. Sensing (S) vs. Intuition (N): This dimension measures how we take in information (perception). The sensing person will rely on the five senses: taste, touch, smell, sight and hearing. The perceptions will be based on inputs from these sources. The intuitive person (N) will not entirely ignore the five senses but rely more heavily on gut feelings or the sixth sense. The person who chooses intuition will describe themselves as innovative while the sensing type will choose to be described as practical. Seventy-five percent of the general population report a preference for sensing (S) while 25% report a preference for intuition (N).

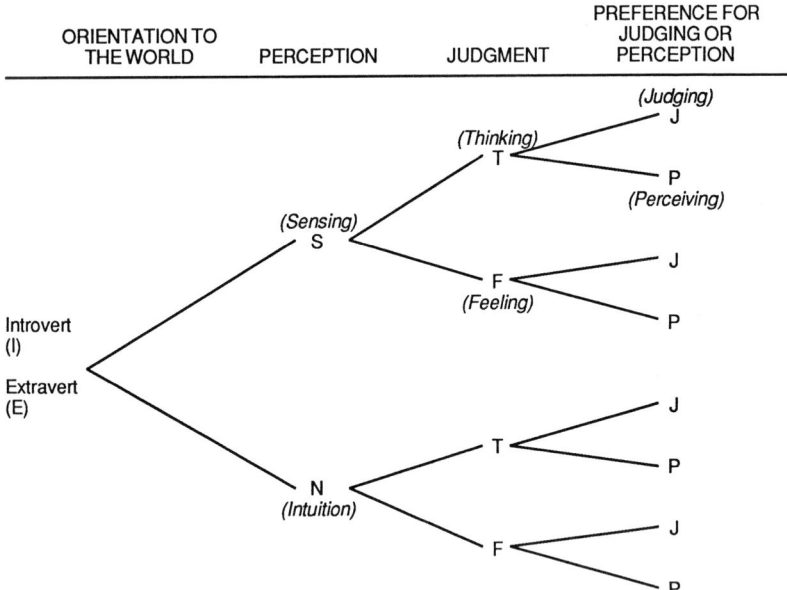

Figure 5.1. Model for Meyer Briggs type indicator (MBTI).

3. __Thinking (T) vs. Feeling (F)__: These preferences describe how we come to conclusions or judgments. When it comes to making a decision, some of us prefer what is called our "thinking" function. We tend to decide things impersonally based upon analysis and principle. People with a thinking preference place a premium on fairness. Some of us will make decisions by valuing alternatives on a personal basis. This is called the "feeling" function. Those of us who have feeling as a preference tend to make decisions and judgments based on liking or disliking, on our values, or on the impact of the decision on people. People with a feeling preference emphasize harmony. The prevalences for the thinking-feeling preferences have slight gender trend: In males, 60% report a preference for thinking (T) and 40% report a preference for feeling (F); in females, 40% report a preference for thinking (T) and 60% report a preference for feeling (F).

4. __Judging (J) vs. Perceiving (P)__: This dimension measures our propensity for closure or openness. Persons who choose closure over open options are likely to be judging types. They are good at planning, organizing, setting deadlines, and reaching a decision. The judging person (J) is apt to report a sense of urgency until a pending decision is reached and then be at rest when the decision is made. The perceiving person (P), in contrast, is more apt to experience resistance to making a decision, wishing more data could be accumulated as the basis for the decision. As a result, when a perceiving person (P) makes a decision, he may have a feeling of uneasiness and restlessness. The prevalence for judging-perceiving preferences are 50% and 50%.

Regardless of the labels of the functions, they have proved to be valuable operational concepts that can differentiate people on the four dimensions. These observable differences among people in action are independent of the label. We will discuss the implications of this psychological assessment tool for intervention purposes.

The MBTI is designed to give a value for each set of preferences, (i.e., a score for both E and I) and a difference score to indicate preference on the dimension. Therefore an individual will have four scores for the four dimensions. These four scores are then combined to form a typology. Given the four scores, 16 types are generated from the assessment. There are great variations within the 16 personality types. The type descriptions initiate self-awareness; they are not the end product. The strength of the assessment is to help people to realize that there are different approaches to perceiving and judging the world. The purpose is self and other awareness to minimize misunderstandings. Many interpersonal conflicts are not over substance but rather style and approach. These style conflicts can get in the way of effective intervention and subsequent behavior change.

Using the Functions for Diagnosis

One of the simplest uses of the MBTI for intervention purposes is to focus on the areas that may need attention. For example:

- Extraverts: Need to listen more and not monopolize discussions
- Introverts: Need to develop assertiveness, influencing skills, and uses of positive power
- Sensing: Need to develop conceptual skills and global focus
- Intuitive: Need to plan more carefully and set realistic objectives
- Thinking: Need to develop more effective interpersonal skills and the ability to give positive, non-critical feedback
- Feeling: Develop the ability to handle criticism
- Judging: Develop skills in stress management
- Perceptives: Develop skills in time management, decision making and planning

The above tags mark the Achilles heel for each individual. The combination of the preferences (four preferences for each person) will, naturally, lead to four areas that we should pay heed to as possible impediments to change. The ESTJ individual (the type more prevalent in the population) will have very different needs than the INFP (a more rare type). The provider should be aware of these needs and use this information in both the design and implementation of the intervention. This methodology is an example of the operational use of the patient/therapist interaction concept. Although an abundant body of literature deals with the patient/therapist interaction, little has been written on the application of these concepts to practice. The MBTI is one assessment that combines a concept with a clinical application. Since the purpose of this chapter is to outline approaches to the effective use of behavioral concepts for intervention, we can not fully develop the theory and application of the MBTI, a project already completed by a number of source books.[19,21] Our intent is to outline some of the uses of psychological assessments to strengthen the intervention design and to prevent bad chemistry in the intervention process.

An Example of the Use of the MBTI in the Design of an Intervention Program

The MBTI can be used to determine the distribution of types in a given intervention program, especially if the design uses group procedures. The most productive approach is to determine the following factors:

- The distribution of extraverts and introverts in the group: This will help the interventionist in balancing discussion time and allow the introverts to be heard during the intervention process.
- The distribution of the four temperament types: Sensing/Judging (SJ), Sensing/Perceiving (SP), Intuitive/Feeling (NF), and Intuitive/Thinking (NT). The usefulness of the types comes not in focusing on all 16 types, but in understanding the temperamental base of the types. The four temperament types have been discussed by such theorists as Jung, Kretschmer, Freud, Adler, Sullivan, and Maslow. Kiersey and Bates[18] have integrated these contributions in a recent book.

The interventionist can use the four temperament types to anticipate what each type appreciates and does not appreciate. This will help eliminate possible misunderstanding between interventionist and participant and between participant and participant. Table 5.2 describes what each temperament type appreciates.

Table 5.2
Appreciation According to Temperament

TEMPERAMENT	WHAT EACH APPRECIATES	WHAT EACH DOES NOT APPRECIATE
Sensing - Judging (SJ) (38% of population)	Praise for task orientation	Deadlines not being met
	Thoroughness, preciseness	Loose procedures
	Want praise but will not show pleasure in receiving it	Meeting not starting and ending on time
Sensing - Perceiving (SP) (38% of population)	Commendation for grace and flair	Being told how to do it
	Process more important than outcome	Standard operating procedures
	Being adaptive and clever	
Intuitive - Feeling (NF) (12% of population)	Personal expressions of praise	Impersonal treatment
	Recognition as a unique person	
	Having feelings and ideas understood by others	
Intuitive - Thinking (NT) (12% of population)	Appreciation for capabilities and ideas	Routine praise out of context
	Someone as competent or more competent appreciating them	Things which violate logic, reason or principle
		Rules, traditions, or biases getting in the way

Implications of the MBTI for Specific Applications

The MBTI helps the interventionist understand personal preferences and the attendant strengths and pitfalls. The MBTI helps us understand how we perceive the world (S or N) and how we judge the world (T or F). A thorough understanding of one's own biases is the first step in eliminating conflict over perception and judgment. For example, an SJ interventionist will design a very different intervention program than either the NT, NF or SP interventionists. The program would fit the preference needs of an all SJ participant group but surely disappoint an SP target group. The MBTI helps the interventionist recognize that meaningful differences among people affect how they perceive and judge. The interventionist can identify compatible and conflicting temperament types. For example, a sensing (S) interventionist would emphasize facts, documentation, careful execution, attention to detail, and practical aspects of the program. An intuitive (N) interventionist would provide the global schema, look for opportunities, indicate challenges, and point out future benefits. The sensing (S) interventionist would work best with the SJ and SP participants but would lose the NT and NF participants. The converse would be true for the intuitive (N) interventionist. The intuitive (N) interventionist would be perceived as too theoretical by most of the general population and must develop a "street smart" sense in dealing with these groups. Table 5.3 points out the interventionist strengths and weaknesses for the four temperament types. They can become checklists for preventing unnecessary conflict over style.

The interventionist should be aware of the distribution of the target group to know how to design the intervention format for the group. Since SJ's and SP's make up 76% of the general population, the probability of their predominating is very high. Of course self-selection may alter these probabilities. The chance of having all NTs or NFs is low. Once the distribution is known, the interventionist may opt to segregate the groups in homogeneous clusters. The design would then be tailored to the needs of that group. Lawrence[20] extensively explores the educational design problems for the SJ and SP student types.

The intervention team should all take the MBTI and hold a weekend retreat to explore their differences and similarities. They then should explore the implications for applying the knowledge to the design of the program, the preferences of the participants, and their intervention style. This can be repeated for maximum effectiveness. Using the MBTI is like learning any skill—it requires practice.

Table 5.3
Interventionist Propensities by temperament

TEMPERAMENT	STRENGTHS	WEAKNESSES
Sensing-Judging (SJ)	Task orientation	Rigidity/inflexibility
	Follows through	Critical
	Well developed procedures	Premature closure
Sensing - Perceiving (SP)	Immediate response to problems	Lack of advance preparation
	Open and flexible style	Lack of follow through
	Strong reality base	Overlooks priorities
Intuitive - Feeling (NF)	Communicates expectations	Creates dependencies
	Is personal, insightful	Too anxious to please
	Allows participation	Moralistic position
Intuitive - Thinking (NT)	Conceptual skills	Escalates standards/ expectations
	Design and innovation	Impatient with feelings/ emotion
	Planning ability	Skepticism

PROBLEM SOLVING APPROACHES TO INTERVENTION

Problem solving approaches (PSA) to intervention are part of the behavioral-cognitive framework. It is one of the key elements in the design that develops responsibility assumption in the participant. The PSA is a method that objectifies the process for both interventionist and participant. The objective of the PSA is to enhance the participant's coping skills. The PSA can be introduced early in the intervention program as a working paradigm for the participant. In order to implement the PSA the following steps should be followed:[22,24,25]

- Define the target behaviors that need to be changed as a problem-to-be-solved.
- Set realistic goals as concretely as possible by stating the problem in behavioral terms and by outlining steps necessary to reach each goal.
- Generate a wide range of possible alternative courses of action.
- Imagine and consider how others might respond if asked to deal with a similar problem.
- Evaluate the pros and cons of each proposed solution and rank order the solutions from least to most practical and desirable.

- Rehearse strategies and behaviors by means of imagery, behavioral rehearsal, and graduated practice.
- Try out the most acceptable and feasible solution.
- Expect some failures, but reward self for having tried.
- Reconsider the original problem in light of the attempt at problem solving.

These steps can be incorporated into a session or sessions especially designed for this purpose. The procedure works best in groups of up to 10 or 12 participants. A productive way to begin the problem-solving process is to ask participants to identify a problem concerning the desired behavior change. Focus on one participant at a time so as to develop the problem. This process can take the following format:

STEPS	QUESTIONS/ACTIONS
Problem Identification	What is involved?
Goal Selection	What do I want?
Generation of Alternatives	What can I do?
Consideration of Consequences	What might happen?
Decision Making	What is my decision?
Implementation	Now do it!
Evaluation	Did it work?

As the procedure progresses, the interventionist may ask for input from other participants in the form of advice, opinion, clarification, and evaluation. This involves them in problem-solving as a group. It always builds the perception that we all face similar dilemmas. The PSA corresponds to overall intervention goals of participant involvement, responsibility assumption, and perceptual change.

CREATING INTERNAL COMMITMENT—SETTING GOALS

Many participants in a health promotion or disease prevention program are unaware of their goals in life. They may never have allowed themselves to focus on what they are trying to achieve. The interventionist should be concerned not only with the specific target behaviors but with the totality of experience of the participants. This involves helping them conceptualize and focus their reasons for existence. Too narrow concern for only target behaviors (i.e., smoking, diet change, exercise program, etc.) may disregard factors in the participants' lives that may interfere with their success in changing the undesired target behaviors. Setting goals has many significant benefits for the participants. For one, it puts them in touch with themselves. Second, it is the first step in taking charge and assuming responsibility for their lives (the sine qua non of intervention objectives). Setting goals prepares the participants mentally and emotionally to set out their commitment to change. The preparation gives them confidence in their ability to meet their needs. The process reinforces the position that they are in charge of their lives. Further, setting goals and working to meet them builds a positive self-image. Finally, the setting of goals provides a focus for their energy and establishes priorities. Therefore, the design of health promotion programs should include a session on goal setting. Again, the range of goals should go beyond just the target behaviors. Some goals may conflict with the desired behavior change and the process may uncover these discrepancies. The participants should be encouraged to include goals that address:

- purpose in life: personal growth, relationships with others, career;
- recreation and relaxation;
- physical activity; and
- specific goals for target behaviors.

The goals in each section should be concrete and specific. As much as possible their abstract goals should be made tangible and objective. In addition to being specific the goals should be measurable. In order to forestall failure, the goals should be realistic and attainable. They should be within the capabilities and life circumstances of the participant. Finally, the goals should be written so that they focus on the partcipant's behavior rather than the hoped-for behavior of others.[25]

The goal setting session should be preceded by a written assignment that takes into account the full range of goals. The next step would be the sharing of goals in small groups or individually with the interventionist and then the setting of action steps. The session should be facilitated by the interventionist, who is a guide through the steps and offers clarification and reinforcement. The follow-through on these goals is presented in the following section on behavioral rehearsal and positive.

RELAXATION TRAINING

Adjunct to Intervention

Unless the intervention program is devoted to stress management, relaxation should be used as an aid to allow the participant to become aware of the messages of the body. Since it is an easy technique to learn, it can be the first step in the program for the participant to gain mastery over stress. Relaxation training can be a daily technique that the participant as an inner resource for encouragement. The specific techniques are basically similar to one another; the interventionist should sample from the full range and choose the technique that suits his or her style.[27,28] Richard Lazarus[29] has produced an excellent audio tape on this subject.

Relaxation training should be introduced as part of the program aimed at getting control of our lives. The interventionist should present the rationale and the objectives of the technique. The main objective is to reduce anxiety and to interrupt the stress-tension cycle that prevents effective performance. The introduction can take the form of a mini-lecture and discussion period. The interventionist should point out that there are many pathways to the relaxation response and the one they are about to experience is only one example.

The second step in the introduction is to understand the expectations of the participants. Some will see it as a game that has little utility. Others may even have the fear that relaxation would be an impediment to performance. It is important to clear up these misperceptions and apprehensions so as to move onto a serious commitment to learning and using the skills.

The third step is to reinforce the need for continued practice and use of the technique for future benefits. The changes will be gradual but cumulative. The objective is to manage stress, not do away with it. In this sense relaxation training becomes an active coping skill.

The next step would be to introduce the relaxation technique using an audio tape and to participate with the group or individual during this session. At the completion of the tape and after the group or individual has relaxed, a discussion of the implications for use in their particular situations would be useful. Then the interventionist can make a bridge between relaxation training and the use of positive imagery as another tool for gaining control.

IMAGERY REHEARSAL

Imagery rehearsal is the process by which an individual can use a skill that we all possess—the ability to imagine events, things, and people in the past, present, and future. We all have the capacity to imagine what happened, is happening and will happen. These images can be accompanied by both positive and negative affect. Exploring what individuals imagine is a clue, sometimes, to whether or not they will be successful in undertaking behavior change. Imagery rehearsal is a specific application to uncovering the blocks and pitfalls in a participant's attempts to change personal behavior.

Imagery rehearsal has been used to help participants to rehearse coping skills or to anticipate future problems. Using imagery rehearsal the participant can approximate real life situations and dilemmas before they occur or reproduce those that have occurred in the past. The use of imagery rehearsal brings into conscious focus the problem, the emotional response, and the means of coping with the situation.[30]

Empirical investigaitons of imagery began with early inquiries into the nature of mental imagery and individual differences in mental imagery capacity. The investigation of mental imagery remained a central part of psychology until about 1920 and then, because of the extreme behavioristic approach in American psychology, it remained a dormant science until the late 1960s. Since that time it has regained a vital place in the experimental and clinical literature.

Meichenbaum[22] has listed all the reasons that can explain why imagery rehearsal works as a clinical intervention. He states that such focusing will:

- help clarify or pinpoint the nature of the participant's current problem;
- reduce unpleasant affect through repetition of the fantasy;
- teach the participant to distinguish between reality and fantasy;
- teach the participant to make finer distinctions among impulsive, motivational, cognitive, and behavioral aspects of the problem;
- teach the participant to control the fantasy scene; and increase the participant's ability to recognize the irrationality of personal beliefs;
- decrease expectancy of disastrous consequences and increase realistic appraisal of external problems;
- make the participant's unconscious conscious.[22]

Meichenbaum states that this cluster of factors helps participants gain increased control over their fantasy lives. In some cases these fantasies or unrealistic thoughts may have paralyzed the participant and caused severe anxiety. By guided imagery rehearsal the participant first begins to understand how he or she influences dysfunctional behavior. Second, this teaches the participant to become aware and to monitor his/her images. Third, the participant becomes in control of their occurrence. Again these are steps in the assumption of responsibility for one's behavior.

Imagery rehearsal can be used with a wide range of behavioral problems and is a nonspecific technique in that sense. It is best used at the implementation stage of the intervention program when the participant is ready to try new behaviors. It can also be used to write new and effective scripts for future performance. An example would be having a participant, through imagery, experience the consequences of going to a party where most people smoked and ate fat laden foods. The individual would be asked to imagine the scene and to anticipate his/her feelings and possible responses to this event. The interventionist would be able to pinpoint possible negative consequences and to have the participant engage in rescripting the outcomes.

An Illustration of Imagery Rehearsal

Meichenbaum[22] notes that the format for imagery rehearsal is derived from Wolpe's[23] Systematic Desensitization Paradigm. The interventionist and the participant collaboratively generate scenarios that could produce stress, concerns or problems related to the desired behavior change. The beginning scenarios should be situations that are easy for the participant to handle. The participant is then asked to imagine coping with progressively more difficult situations while relaxed. Then the participant is asked to imagine coping with the difficult situation. The goal is to have the participant learn to notice, even anticipate, signs of distress, so that these become cues that produce coping responses. At this stage the use of coping imagery involves the participants' imagining themselves becoming distressed, having associated thoughts and feelings, and then generating coping responses. In some instances the participant may have to generate a new approach to the situation by acquiring, under guidance, different coping skills. This is all part of the treatment regime. The participant is encouraged to use any personally generated statements and images that would enhance coping. Since the procedure starts out with easy transactions, the participant can go back to these coping scenes if coping with more stressful events proves difficult. In this context, imagery rehearsal can help the participant to identify pitfalls, anticipate emotional responses, and objectify new behaviors.

Imagery rehearsal is only one behavioral technique that should be integrated within the design of the overall intervention program. It is not an end in itself but a pathway to help the participant gain control over the situation. Since imagery rehearsal has had successful applications in weight loss, smoking cessation, and stress reduction programs, the relevance to health maintenance programs as an adjunct technique should be explored.

BEHAVIORAL REHEARSAL

Behavioral rehearsal has been defined by Lazarus[31] as "a specific procedure which aims to replace deficient interpersonal responses by efficient and effective behavior patterns. The patient achieves this by practicing the desired forms of behavior under the direction and supervision of the therapist." In actuality, this process is an elaboration of Moreno's[32] early "psychodrama" technique. In both situations the participants are asked to play a role and to act out either their normal responses or new coping behaviors. Janis and Mann[33] have validated the successful use of behavioral rehearsal in smoking cessation programs. Their findings support Bandura's[34] contention that the participant should be actively involved in constructing new coping behaviors. The implementation of the behavioral rehearsal procedure usually involves the following steps:

- the specification of the problem and identification of specific behaviors to be acquired for effective performance;
- the interventionist, acting as participant, models specific behaviors in a simulated situation;
- discussion of the modeled behavior;
- simulation of the situation this time with the participant practicing the desired behavior;
- the interventionist giving feedback about the "performance";
- carrying out the new role in real life;
- evaluation by interventionist and participant of real life performance.

Behavioral rehearsal is easy to implement and provides the participant an active role in the intervention process. This procedure can be used in conjunction with the other techniques discussed in this chapter.[31-36]

SUMMARY

One can anticipate a high degree of success with the highly motivated, low-risk participants, but one must be innovative and highly motivated to deal with the stressed, high-risk participants. The high-risk participant offers the greatest payoffs for risk reduction and reduced morbidity and mortality. This chapter has presented a conceptual and practical framework for approaching problems of behavior change in the design and execution of preventive health care programs based on the assumptions that there are no simple solutions to difficult problems and that the designers and facilitators of preventive programs must assess the strengths and weaknesses o the target population to determine the appropriate strategies and techniques. The array of behavioral methodologies presented in this chapter have demonstrated validities for dealing with problems of smoking cessation, stress management, nutrition modification, and medication compliance. See Appendix 5-1 for an outline of a ten session program to nutrition modification. In addition to the application of behavioral techniques, the roles of the facilitator and the participant are critical factors in determining the success or failure of the program. The development of an explicit psychological contract between the facilitator and the participant is the first step in building responsibility assumption on the part of the participant.

REFERENCES

1. Benfari RC, Eaker E, Stroll JG: Behavioral interventions and compliance to treatment regimes. Ann Rev Public Health 1981;2: 431-471.

2. Sackett DL, Haynes RB: Compliance with Therapeutic Regimens. Baltimore, MD: John Hopkins Press, 1976.

3. Weinstein M, Stason WB: Hypertension: Applying Perspective. Cambridge, MA: Harvard University Press, 1976.

4. Ockene JK, Hymowitz N, Sexton M, Broste SB: Comparison of patterns of smoking behavior change among smokers in the Multiple Risk Factor Intervention Trial (MRFIT). Prev Med 1981;10:621-638.

5. Multiple Risk Factor Intervention Trial Research Group: Risk factor changes and mortality results: MRFIT. JAMA 1982;248:1465-1477.

6. Baric L: Recognition of the at-risk role. Internat J Health Educ 1969;12:35-44.

7. Benfari RC: The Multiple Risk Factor Intervention Trial (MRFIT). II. The model for intervention. Prev Med 1981;10:426-442.

8. Yalom I: Existental Psychotherapy. New York: Basic Books, 1980: 231-253.

9. Argyris C: Increasing Leadership Effectiveness. New York: John Wiley, 1976.

10. White RW: Motivation reconsidered: The concept of competence. Psych Rev 1959:297-333.

11. Kelman HC: Processes of opinion change. Pub Opin Quarter 1961;25: 57-78.

12. Luborsky L: Principles of Psychoanalytic Psychotherapy: a Manual for Supportive-Expressive Treatment. New York: Basic Books, 1984.

13. Rotter JB: Generalized expectancies for internal versus external control of reinforcement. Psychological Monograph 1966;80:609.

14. Ellis: Reason and emotion in psychotherapy. New York: Lyle Stuart, 1962.

15. Lazarus R: Behavior Therapy and Beyond. New York: McGraw Hill, 1971.

16. Goldfried MR, DeCentecco ET, Weinberg L: Systematic rational restructuring as a self-control technique. Behav Ther 1974;5: 247-254.

17. Stuart R: Behavior contracting within the families of delinquents. J Behavior Ther and Exper Psychiat 1971;2:1-11.

18. MBTI. Palo Alto, CA: Consulting Psychologists Press, Inc., 1977.

19. Kiersey D and Bates M: Please Understand Me. Del Mar, CA: Prometheus Nemesis Books, 1978.

20. Lawrence G: People Types and Tiger Stripes (ed. 2). Gainesville, FL: Center for Applications of Psychological Type (CAPT), Inc., 1979.

20a. Quenk AT and Quenk NL: The use of psychological typologies in analysis. IN: Stein M (ed): Jungian Analysis. Boston: New Science Library, 1984.

21. Krebs SH: Using the Meyers-Briggs Type Indicator in Organizations: A Resource Book. Palo Alto, CA: Consulting Psychologists Press Inc., 1985.

22. Meichenbaum D: Stress Inoculation Training. New York: Pergamon Press, 1985.

23. Wolpe J: Psychotherapy by Reciprocal Inhibition. Stanford, CA: Stanford University Press, 1959.

24. Beck A: Cognitive Approaches to Stress. IN: Woolfolk R and Lehrer P (eds.): Principles and Practice of Stress Management. New York: Guilford Press, 1984.

25. D'Zurilla J and Nezu A: Social Problem-Solving in Adults. IN: Kendall D (ed.): Advances in Cognitive-behavioral Research and Therapy (Vol. 1). New York: Academic Press, 1982.

26. Sobel H and Wordan J: Helping Cancer Patients Cope: A Problem-Solving Intervention for Health Care Professionals. New York: Guilford Press, 1981.

27. Woolfolk R and Lehrer P: Principles and Practice of Stress Management. New York: Guilford Press, 1984.

28. Benson H: The Relaxation Response. New York: William Morrow, 1975.

29. Lazarus A: Relaxation I & II (audio tape). Chicago: Instructional Development Inc., 1970.

30. McCaffery M: Nursing Management of the Patient with Pain. Philadelphia: JB Lippincott, 1979.

31. Lazarus A: Behavior rehearsal vs non-directive therapy vs advice in effective behavior change. Behav Res Ther 1966;4:209-212.

32. Moreno JL: Psychodrama. New York: Beacon Press, 1946.

33. Janis I and Mann L: Effectiveness of emotional role playing on desire to modify smoking habits and attitudes. Internat Exper Res Perspect 1965;7:17-27.

34. Bandura A: Self-efficacy: Toward a unifying theory of behavior change. Psychol Rev 1977;84:191-205.

35. Wolpe J: Psychotherapy by Reciprocal Inhibition. Stanford, CA: Stanford University Press, 1959.

36. Turk D, Meichenbaum D and Benest M: Pain and Behavioral Medicine. New York: Guilford Press, 1959.

37. West D, Horan J and Eames P: Component analysis of occupational stress inoculation applied to registered nurses in an acute care hospital setting. J Counsel Psychol 1984;31:209-218.

Appendix 5.1
Ten Session Group Program for Clients Who Want to Modify Their Eating Behavior

OPENING SESSION 1

The problem; epidemiological data
The rationale for intervention
Personal relevance
Expectations
Roles
Discussion
Assignment for next session (Meyer-Briggs and Rotter forms)

SESSION 2

Presentation of the food pattern
Feedback on food records
Group discussion of food patterns in the group
Participant identification of targeted changes

SESSION 3

Feedback and interpretation of MBTI and Rotter
What it means for personal change: pitfalls and pathways
Small group discussion of results -- facilitator led

SESSION 4

Contracting for change
Identification of problems and difficulties
Discussion of ways to cope
Handout food record II

SESSION 5

Behavioral rehearsal
Role plays
Feedback and discussion -- facilitator led

SESSION 6

Feedback on second food record
Pinpointing of successes and failures
Relaxation introduced
Role of stress reduction in the intervention program

SESSION 7

Problem identification
Imagery introduced and practiced
Discussion

Appendix 5.1 (Cont'd.)
Ten Session Group Program for Clients Who Want to Modify Their Eating Behavior

SESSION 8

Presentation of new ways of food preparation
Films
Discussion
Contracting revisited

SESSION 9

Imagery and behavioral rehearsal II
Discussion of problem areas

SESSION 10

Responsibility assumption revisited
Problems encountered
Contracting for the future

CHAPTER 6

Practice Management for Clinical Prevention
G. Frederick Vanderschmidt, Ph.D.

Every medical practice has a system of management. The system may be explicit, represented by written operating procedures and organization charts. It may be implicit, represented by "do it this way" conversations between members of the practice. This chapter deals with the special management problems which a practice must consider when undertaking preventive initiatives. Such initiatives pose the following special management questions:

- What kind of preventive initiatives require modification of the practice's management?
- How should such preventive initiatives be organized?
- How do such preventive initiatives generate income?
- What are the record keeping requirements for preventive initiatives?

KINDS OF PRACTICE

Management ideas must relate to the kind of practice involved. Three types of practice are usual: solo practice, group practice, and institutional practice. In the following sections of this chapter some suggestions are made relating to one or another of these practice types. As the following discussion suggests, sometimes it's difficult to characterize a practice as one of these types.

What Kind of a Practice?

John Brady is an internist with an office in a city in the San Joaquin Valley of California. His office is attached to his house; he employs a receptionist/bookkeeper, Ms. Alsop, who answers the telephone and takes care of office business. In the past Dr. Brady described his practice as a solo practice. However, two years ago the county medical society organized a health maintenance organization (HMO) along the lines of a foundation for health care or independent practice association. The foundation organized most of the private primary care practices in the county, including Dr. Brady's, to function as a kind of HMO without walls. The foundation offers local employers a health care plan which, on the basis of a fixed

annual premium, guarantees that all the medical care needs of
their employees will be covered, using any foundation practitioner chosen by the employee. Since the foundation qualifies
as an HMO under federal definition, local employers must offer
its services as an alternative (there is no other local HMO in
the area).

The foundation's practitioners, like Dr. Brady, are paid
by the foundation for treating subscribers to the foundation's
service according to an interim schedule of fees not too different from those charged by Dr. Brady to other patients using
his practice. Any surplus of premium over outlay is distributed to the member practices at the end of the year as a
bonus; should the premiums not cover the total paid for services, the amount paid to the practices is reduced the
following year to make up the deficit.

Dr. Brady notes that HMOs are often cited as examples of
institutional practice. Dr. Brady also recalls that a friend
described the foundation as "essentially a large group
practice." So, although he still thinks of himself as a solo
practice, he isn't so sure that others would see him in that
light because of his involvement with the foundation.

*   *   *

With respect to management, the type of practice can be determined
by comparison with the profiles shown in Table 6.1. In spite of Dr.
Brady's association with the foundation, he would find himself best
described by the "solo" profile. The profiles do not represent the only
ways to practice or the best ways to practice; few practices will fit
any profile exactly. For instance, the profile for group practice
assumes a group of physician entrepreneurs; in fact, the entrepreneurial
group may include nonphysicians such as nurse practitioners (so called
"collaborative" practice). A nurse practitioner may even establish a
solo practice without affiliation with physicians. However, most practices will identify closely with one of the three profiles.

PREVENTIVE INITIATIVES

Most practices provide some preventive medicine and have organized a
management approach which accommodates these initiatives. "Secondary
prevention," that is the early detection of asymptomatic disease, fits
readily into established management systems since such prevention is
closely associated with the tradition of treatment of acute, symptomatic
disease. "Primary prevention," that is the reduction of risk of a
disease, is less likely to fit into established management systems.
Although some forms of primary prevention such as immunization have been
accommodated, others -- particularly those requiring the modification of
the patient's life style -- are likely to require changes in the
management of the practice. In particular, they often require the use
of personnel and outside facilities not normally used by the practice,

Table 6.1
Profiles of Three Types of Practice

PROFILE ELEMENT	SOLO PRACTICE	GROUP PRACTICE	INSTITUTIONAL PRACTICE
What is the relation between the physician(s) and the practice?	Only one physician associated with the practice	Several physicians are associated with the practice, sharing facilities and personnel	A number of physicians are salaried employees of the institution
Why do patients use the practice?	Patients come to the practice because of the physician's specialty and reputation	Patients come to the practice because of the specialty and reputation of one of the physicians in the group	Patients come to the practice because of the reputation of the institution, because of special service available through the institution, or because the cost is low or free
Who treats the patients?	Most treatment is provided by the physician	Most treatment is provided by one of the group's physicians. Greater use is made of non-physician practitioners than in solo practice	Considerable use is made of non-physician practitioners
How are patients referred to other specialties?	Patients are referred outside the practice	Patients are referred within the practice if possible	Patients are referred within the practice
Who is responsible for the practice?	The physician	The physician group. The group may delegate this responsibility to an employee administrator	A chief administrator reporting to a board of directors, trustees, or government authority

Table 6.1 (Cont'd.)
Profiles of Three Types of Practice

PROFILE ELEMENT	SOLO PRACTICE	GROUP PRACTICE	INSTITUTIONAL PRACTICE
Who is responsible for the quality of the services provided?	The physician	Each physician in the group has autonomy in the care provided to his patients. Some informal interaction occurs among members of the group on quality issues	Patient treatment often scrutinized by physician and nonphysician personnel other than physician initially responsible for the patient
How are the physicians compensated?	Excess of practice income over expense	Excess of practice income over expense, shared on the basis of a formula agreed upon by the group	Salary paid by the institution
What is the relation of nonphysician personnel to the practice?	Salaried by or contracted to practice; accountable to the physician	Salaried by or contracted to practice; accountable to the physicians, sometimes through an administrator	Salaried by or contracted to the practice; a hierarchy of physicians, nonphysician practitioners, and administrators exists with complex, interrelated lines of authority and accountability

the development of reimbursement approaches not normally used by the practice, and the development of information systems not normally used by the practice. This chapter deals with these issues.

Examples of preventive initiatives which are likely to require significant changes in a traditional practice's management include:

- Smoking Cessation. A patient who stops smoking will substantially reduce the risk of cancer of the lung, heart disease, and other diseases; women who stop smoking in pregnancy will have children with higher birth weight. Smoking cessation programs involve approaches not common in the practice of acute medicine.

- **Hypertension.** Control of hypertension reduces the risk of heart disease. Although control of hypertension is often an initiative undertaken by a practice, an aggressive program may well affect the management of the practice, particularly a program which stresses weight control, salt restriction, and exercise as alternatives or aid to a pharmacological approach.

- **Cholesterol.** Reduction of the level of cholesterol in the patient's blood serum reduces the risk of heart disease; such control usually involves changing the patient's dietary habits.

Other preventive initiatives which require changes in the traditional practice's management include weight control, control of alcohol and drug abuse, control of workplace exposures, and stress control; a more complete listing will be found in Chapter 3.

Logically a practice should concern itself with any preventive initiative with some scientific basis (see Chapter 2). These initiatives have often been combined into age- and sex-specific packages as described in Chapter 3. There are, however, limitations on the preventive initiatives which a practice can undertake.

In reviewing preventive initiatives, two factors bear upon the practice setting. First, the specialty of the practice must be considered. Most of the initiatives described in Chapter 3 are applicable to the practice of primary care with emphasis on an adult patient population. Second, the initiatives involve the organization of resources beyond the traditional physician/patient interaction. In group practice and institutional practice, other members of the practice must be involved in making the decision to organize these resources and to accept the redirection of their time required by the preventive initiatives introduced.

Finally, in any kind of practice, initiative involves financial risk. The amount of risk which the practice is willing to accept at any time will have some limits (see the section on "Income" in this chapter).

An example of the way in which a practice takes on a preventive initiative which will involve significant changes in the practice management is provided by the example of Dr. Warren Pratt. Each practice will approach the decisions involved in clinical prevention in a different way; the group practice with which Dr. Pratt is associated is no exception.

Taking on a Preventive Initiative

Dr. Warren Pratt began his practice in internal medicine ten years ago as a solo practitioner. He has always been interested in the emotional health of his patients and in preventive medicine. Dr. Pratt now has four physician partners; the practice also employs two registered nurses. Together these practitioners have incorporated preventive assessments into their protocols for seeing patients. Much of this assessment has been the responsibility of the two RNs, Ms. Aycock and Ms. Spann, who initially see each patient before the physician.

Recently the group has been considering how the practice could address disease prevention and health promotion in a more aggressive manner. The group agrees to adopt a preventive initiative on a trial basis during which they will determine how well the initiative is working and whether it can pay for itself. If the group feels that the initiative is successful after a year of experience, they will consider other preventive initiatives. Dr. Pratt and Ms. Aycock volunteer to plan the implementation process.

Accepting the limitation of a single initiative, Dr. Pratt and Ms. Aycock are eager to maximize the success of the trial. It seems to Dr. Pratt that most of the initiatives described in Chapter 3 relate to conditions and populations with which the practice is concerned. However, Ms. Aycock relates that several of the initiatives are addressed by existing community services; for instance, she has high regard for local substance abuse programs and for a weight control clinic operated by a local hospital.

Both Ms. Aycock and Dr. Pratt believe an effective smoking cessation program would involve a group of about ten patients. The practice has no suitable meeting space for such a group, so they decide to eliminate smoking control from consideration.

Of the remaining initiatives, Dr. Pratt's longstanding personal interest in emotional health is rekindled. The practice is located in a recently developed suburban area whose largest employers are manufacturing concerns. Reductions have been made in the number of hours for which office staff at these plants are paid and nearly one quarter of the firms' line workers have been laid off. Both Ms. Aycock and Ms. Spann have noted an increase in stress related complaints and disorders among patients, including a few suspected cases of child abuse. To obtain objective data the office assistant is asked to review a sample of the practice's preventive assessments.

The assistant reports back that of several hundred assessments reviewed from patients coming in the last few months:

- Approximately 17 percent of the adults assessed reported too much fighting with spouses and children.

128 HANDBOOK OF CLINICAL PREVENTION

- Some 10 percent of the adult males presented ulcer or colitis-like conditions or other conditions associated with stress.
- The incidence of complaints of sexual problems seemed to be rising.
- There appeared to be an increasing number of visits where other stress related problems were presented.

Dr. Pratt and Ms. Aycock decide a preventive program in stress control should be offered as the practice's first initiative. The method for making the choice is a rather complex mixture of objective considerations and subjective interests, supported by some evidence from the practice.

ORGANIZING PREVENTIVE INITIATIVES BY DEVELOPING PROTOCOLS

In dealing with a patient, a practitioner always has some general scheme in mind, even though the scheme may not be explicit and may encompass a number of alternatives. Such schemes are called protocols. There are advantages to making such schemes explicit, however. An explicit protocol allows the identification and organization of personnel and community resources to help the practitioner meet patient needs; an explicit protocol allows organization of an effective information system. Explicit protocols do not take the place of professional judgment; they identify the points in the patient/practice relationship where such judgment must be made.

In this section the description of a protocol using a flow chart is suggested. Flow charting provides a simple, graphic method for presenting protocols. Complex protocols can be described by breaking down the overall protocol into smaller parts, each of which can then be represented by a reasonably simple flow chart. For a complete exposition of flow charting one of the older books on data processing is suggested.[1]

In his book *Preventive Primary Medicine*[2] Dr. Robert Lewy makes the point, "Much of the material covered in this book remains controversial. There is no universally accepted preventive health protocol." Thus the substance of any protocol used by a practice will usually have some basis in the experience of the professionals in the practice and some basis in the published work which exists. The protocol will change as the practice's experience with it grows and as other information becomes available from other workers.

To develop a protocol flow chart take the following steps.

Step 1. *Identify the procedure covered by the protocol.* Protocol flow charts are useful when a patient is identified as a candidate for intervention to reduce a risk factor. Good examples include the risk factors for heart disease: smoking, hypertension, and hypercholesterolemia. Be exact in identifying the procedure to be flow charted.

Good example: how to deal with a patient who smokes. (A specific, manageable problem.)

Poor example: how to practice preventive medicine. (Too large a topic; not clear what is encompassed.)

Step 2. Decide at what point the procedure begins and ends. Any flow chart begins at the "enter" point, that is, the point at which the procedure begins, and finishes at one or more "exit" points which represent the possible conclusions of the process.

The exit points of the procedure should represent the desired goal of the procedure and any other logical occurrence which ends the procedure. Thus the exit points for a procedure dealing with smoking cessation should include permanent smoking cessation and also the possibility that the patient drops out of the program for various reasons (patient rejects treatment, moves away, dies).

Step 3. Chart actions and decisions leading from the entrance to the exit(s) of the flow chart. Use rectangular boxes to describe actions and diamond shaped boxes to describe decisions. Connect the rectangles and diamonds together with arrows which describe the logical flow of the procedure. Most flow charts will have two important characteristics: branching and looping.

- Any diamond shaped decision box indicates a choice. Such boxes will have two (or more) arrows proceeding from them, depending on which decision is made. Such a pattern is called a "branch."

- Often certain activities will be repeated over and over. Such repetitive patterns are established by showing an arrow leading from the last box in the activity pattern back to the first box. Such a pattern is called a "loop."

A protocol flow chart is a tool to organize a process which may involve the help of other people and the support of an information system; it's not an end in itself. Flow charts should help organize and communicate. If the thought is simple enough to organize and communicate without a flow chart, don't make one. If you feel more comfortable organizing and communicating a process in some other format, use it.[3]

The flow chart approach is very flexible; one can develop a flow chart in such detail that it is applicable only to a particular practice, or approach the matter in such a general way that the flow chart could be applied to any type of practice providing primary care. For an example, we will take the general way as shown in the protocol flow chart of Figure 6.1.

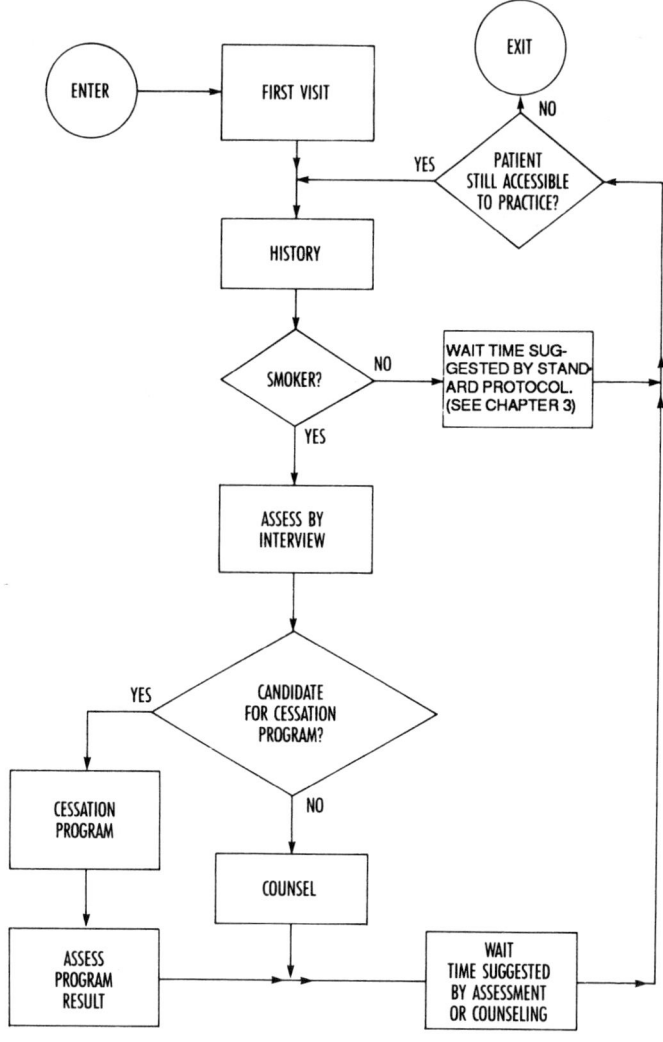

Figure 6.1. A flow chart describing the protocol for a smoking cessation program. The chart is sufficiently general to apply to almost any practice setting providing primary care to adults.

A Smoking Cessation Protocol Flow Chart

Step 1. Identify the procedure to be covered by the protocol. The procedure in this example is to be followed by the practice to control the smoking risk factor of all patients associated with the practice.

Step 2. Decide at what point the procedure begins and ends. For our example, let us assume that the procedure begins at the point where a patient first comes to the practice. As a part of the history taken at this point, the questions "do you smoke?" is asked, without further elaboration.

Following the recommended practice for controlling smoking as described in Chapter 4, the practice continues to assess the patient and attempts to eliminate smoking behavior as long as the patient is associated with the practice; thus the procedure ends only when this association ends.

Step 3. Chart the actions and decisions leading from the entrance to the exit of the flow chart. Following the initial history, smokers and nonsmokers can be identified. Nonsmokers require no intervention, but should be followed at regular intervals to make sure they have not started smoking. This repetitive followup introduces a loop in the flow pattern which is broken only when the patient is no longer accessible to the practice.

Smokers are interviewed at greater length about their smoking habit, irrespective of the complaint which brought them to the practice, but usually concurrently with a discussion of the complaint (whether or not the smoking behavior is germane to the complaint). The purpose is to assess how serious the risk is for the patient and to gain some insight into what kind of smoking cessation approach might work with the patient.

At this point we assume that the practice has access to formal smoking cessation programs. One or more of the programs may be offered by the practice itself. Other programs may be used when the practice believes them sound and when they provide the practice with information about the progress of the patient. On the basis of the interview and the assessment, a decision is made whether or not to recommend participation in one of the formal smoking cessation programs.

The following are reasons for not placing a patient in such a program:

- The patient refuses to cooperate. ("I can't stop smoking, and, to tell you the truth, I don't want to; I'll take my chances with the risks.")

- The patient's habit is very mild; the time and expense of the formal program seem inappropriate. (An 80-year-old woman smokes a single cigarette after dinner.)

- The patient cannot afford the expense of the program, and no "scholarship" assistance is available; no free community program is available.

- The patient has been through a cessation program without notable improvement.

Such patients are provided with whatever ad hoc counseling the practice can afford; the others are placed in one of the cessation programs.

Patients who are placed in a cessation program are monitored; at the conclusion of the program, their progress is assessed by feedback from the program staff. Depending on the cessation program result or the ad hoc counseling (whichever branch the patient has taken) a follow-up time is scheduled and the process begins again.

STAFFING PREVENTIVE INITIATIVES

Each of the boxes on the flow chart describes an activity or a decision to be made. The manager is now to decide who will be responsible for each activity and decision. Further, a decision must be made on some of the activities: Will the activity be undertaken by the practice or will the patient be referred (with suitable control) to an outside practice or agency?

Certain tasks involving the assessment and monitoring of the patient's progress belong within the practice itself. Interventions requiring resources which the practice does not have may require referral if such resources are available in the community. Examples of such referral are the use of a smoking cessation program offered by a local branch of the American Heart Association or the use of a weight control program offered by a local hospital clinic.

First, however, consider the personnel which the practice has or may wish to acquire (possibly on a part-time basis) in order to run its own programs. At least the following categories of individuals should be considered in making staffing decisions.[4]

Physicians. The use of physicians as personnel in preventive initiatives should be considered in the context of certain assets and liabilities. Among the assets is the authority represented by the physician, often a powerful motivating influence. Further, protocols for preventive initiatives often require one or more assessments of the patient which are convenient to combine with the physician's examination of the patient for other problems.

On the other hand, physician time is expensive. In addition, there is a need for motivation beyond that represented by the physician's authority. Such motivation is an important problem in primary prevention. Some physicians are interested in this problem and do a good job; others are not interested and thus do not perform well.

Nurses. Nursing education, particularly advanced training in the area of primary care leading to nurse practitioner status, often encourages close, individual concern with the patient; further, nurses have the clinical skill to handle history taking and other assessment and intervention procedures.[5,6] The amount of experience with specific preventive initiatives will vary.

Physician Assistants. A number of training programs exist for providing personnel with some medical care skills in a program which is on a different track from nursing education. It is difficult to generalize about how well such individuals might fit into a preventive initiative; as with nurses, they may be effective in history taking and other assessment procedures, and, depending on their training and interests, in the intervention process.

Clinical Psychologists. Individuals trained in clinical psychology are usually interested and knowledgeable about the problems and possibilities of counseling. They may or may not be knowledgeable about the preventive initiatives which the practice wishes to implement.

Health Educators. Individuals trained in the area of health education are often knowledgeable about preventive initiatives. They may or may not have had "hands on" experience in counseling patients.

Nutritionists. Nutritionists are always knowledgeable about preventive initiatives which are affected by diet; they have good skills on the technical side of the problem. Their skill in counseling patients depends on the background and the attitude of the individual.

Secretary Receptionist. The secretary receptionist is often a very useful member of the preventive initiative group, particularly in managing the information system aspects of the initiative.

The assignment of personnel to specific activities required by the protocol involves the delegation of authority. The manager must understand the position of each individual within the organization and the activities which can be appropriately delegated to each individual from an operational and -- to some extent -- a legal point of view.

The most obvious factors which relate to practice setting are, first, the size of the practice and, second, whether it is in a rural or an urban setting.

Large practices, particularly those which are institutional in nature, will have many of the resources needed to set up programs. Nutritionists, psychologists, nurse practitioners, and health educators already may be on the staff; to the extent that these personnel are available, they represent resources which may be used to implement preventive initiatives. Once the manager has convinced the appropriate decision makers to support the initiative, the availability of such internal resources often simplifies implementation.

A more difficult task is faced by solo and group practices, particularly those located in rural areas. Such practices are likely to be small with limited internal resources to draw upon, and the pool of appropriate personnel in the community may be limited. Such practices must recruit aggressively and use resources which may not always be ideal for the initiative's activities.

A Practice-Staffed Preventive Initiative in Smoking Cessation

Dr. Peter Schmidt is an internist; he has also trained as a subspecialist in the field of rheumatology. After working for a number of years as a member of a group practice using the facilities of a small hospital specializing in the field of rheumatology, he decided to set up an independent practice. He now works in a condominium office which he owns on a well traveled street in a well-to-do neighborhood on the outskirts of the city. There are two small offices: one for Dr. Schmidt and one for Kathryn Doyle, a nurse practitioner. They share the two examination rooms and a utility room. Besides Ms. Doyle, Dr. Schmidt employs a secretary/receptionist.

Recently Ms. Doyle and Dr. Schmidt have become interested in establishing an organized program of preventive medicine within the practice. Reviewing the practice, they characterize their patients' main risk factor as smoking. Both Dr. Schmidt and Ms. Doyle have been impressed with the success of the MRFIT program in achieving a marked reduction in the smoking behavior of a group of men whose age is in the same range as many of their own patients (see Figure 6.2).

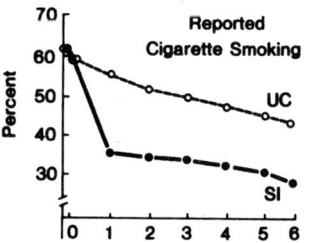 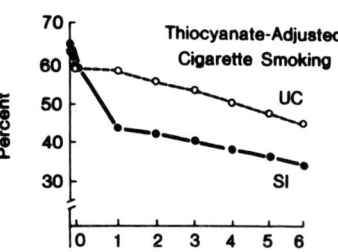

<u>Figure 6.2.</u> Decline in smoking as observed by patients participating in MRFIT. The more rapid decline was among individuals subjected to intensive intervention (SI); the less rapid decline occurred among individuals with conventional intervention (UC). The horizontal axis is years.

Dr. Schmidt and Ms. Doyle choose a protocol which can be described by the flow chart in Figure 6.1 and decide to establish within their own practice a cessation program similar to the MRFIT program in which small groups of patients were counseled by a MRFIT staff member. These sessions occurred weekly for approximately ten weeks. Table 6.2 outlines the assignment of personnel for this program.

Table 6.2
Assignment of Personnel for Smoking Cessation Protocol

ACTIVITY/DECISION (See Figure 6.1)	RESPONSIBLE	COMMENT
First visit	Secretary/receptionist	Requires scheduling
History	Nurse practitioner	This person normally takes the history required of all patients and performs a physical examination
Smoker?	Nurse practitioner	Decision based on history
Assess smokers by interview	Physician	Assessment made as a part of the interview covering all aspects of the patient's visit
Candidate for cessation program?	Physician	Decision based on basis of assessment interview
Cessation program	Clinical psychologist	This person must be recruited by the practice. Should be experienced with this type of program
Assess program result	Clinical psychologist	
Counsel	Physician	Counseling is provided at assessment interview
Decide on time to wait before recontracting patient	Clinical psychologist or physician	Person responsible depends on whether patient was in cessation program branch or counseling branch
Patient still accessible to practice?	Secretary/receptionist	

136 HANDBOOK OF CLINICAL PREVENTION

USING COMMUNITY RESOURCES

When making decisions about a preventive initiative, the manager will often consider using an intervention outside of the practice for some phase of the protocol. Such resources may be available through the health care establishment, through volunteer organizations, or through commercial establishments; we refer to them as community resources.

Referral of a patient to an outside intervention does not imply that the practice loses control of the patient. In the context of the preventive initiative such referrals are similar to sending a patient to another doctor for an X ray or a laboratory test. The referring practice expects the service to be performed promptly and expertly and the results of the service to be communicated directly to the practice.

A practice might wish to refer a patient to an outside service for a number of reasons. The practice may not be able to afford to set up its own smoking cessation program or weight loss program. If the practice does set up its own program, the approach adapted by the practice may not be effective for all of the practice's patients; alternative programs available from community resources may be desirable.

The option to refer patients to services offered by community resources is most likely to concern the manager of a small practice since the risk of establishing an internal program may be too great. If such a practice is located in an urban setting, community resources will abound (although their quality will vary widely). Practices in rural settings may have difficulty finding appropriate community resources.

The following steps should be taken to use community resources.

Step 1. Identify available community resources. The protocol developed for a particular preventive initiative will contain one or more interventions for which the manager may wish to use community resources. Locating such resources is accomplished by using a variety of information sources. These contacts are asked to provide information on suitable services available in the community and to suggest other sources of information. This "networking" process will usually promptly identify community resources for a well defined preventive initiative.

In some cases a licensure requirement will allow the use of licensing authority listing. In some cases voluntary organizations or departments or public health will have developed listings.

Step 2. Evaluate identified services. Before making a community resource a part of the preventive initiative's protocol, the manager should be sure that the intervention has a reasonable chance of success. Some member of the practice should talk with the staff of the resource and, if possible, attend sessions between patient and resource staff. Two important factors which should be explored with the resource are the cost to the patient and the kind of information which the practice can obtain from the resource on the progress of the patient in the resources's program.

Step 3. Make Arrangements With the Community Resource. If, at the conclusion of Step 2, a decision is made to employ an intervention offered by a community resource in a practice's preventive initiative, a working arrangement should be made between the practice and the community resource. The agreement should define the practice's intention to refer a certain number of patients for certain services at a certain cost to the patient, with certain information to be provided the practice on the patient's progress. Such arrangements should be made clear in a written agreement between the practice and the community resource.

Using Community Resources

Mary Kelly is a pediatric nurse practitioner who manages the maternal and child health clinic at city hospital. The clinic provides primary care for low income city residents in the area of pregnancy, birth, and child care. Some of the clinic's patients have insurance (many are covered by Medicaid) which covers the clinic's services; some make a nominal payment out of pocket based on a "sliding scale." The clinic also receives support from the federal government and from the city to help cover the operating deficit.

The clinic has decided to embark upon a systematic program for eliminating smoking among the pregnant women and young mothers who, along with their children, are the clinic's patients. The initiative seems particularly important because of growing evidence that smoking during pregnancy is associated with low birth weight among infants. Further, Ms. Kelly believes that a parent's smoking habit can't be a good example to set for children.

However, budgets are very tight. Even though the city hospital could staff a smoking cessation program completely, using employees and consultants, the decision has been made for the moment to find an outside resource in the community in order to implement the box labeled "cessation program" in the flow chart of Figure 6.1. The other requirements of the flow chart can be met within budget constraints by the clinic staff. Thus Ms. Kelly has the job of locating a suitable cessation program to which patients who are judged candidates can be referred.

The task of finding a professionally acceptable program is made more difficult by two additional problems. Most of the clinic's patients cannot afford a program which costs more than a few dollars. Further, because the hospital is funded from public sources, referrals must not show any favoritism among potential suppliers. Ms. Kelly will have to refer patients to any program which can meet reasonable criteria.

Ms. Kelly begins with Step 1 as described above (identify available community resources). Using spare moments in her busy schedule, Ms. Kelly makes some phone calls over a week's time to learn something about smoking cessation programs. She starts out by looking in the telephone directory Yellow Pages under "smoking;" she finds a listing category "smokers information and treatment centers." She eliminates some of the listings; although she hasn't yet developed a formal list of criteria which a program should fulfill, she thinks it unlikely that the "Acupuncture Stop Smoking Clinic" or programs which use hypnosis would be acceptable. She phones the remaining listings: two licensed psychologists, a private clinic, and a self help group; she is able to elicit a brief description of each program and its cost.

Searching further, Ms. Kelly looks in the Yellow Pages under "Social Service Organizations." Here she finds listings for the local chapters of the American Cancer Society and American Lung Association. Calls to these offices elicit descriptions of programs; further she is referred to the state Cancer Information Service (available in every state) which maintains a list of smoking cessation programs available throughout the state. Using this list and other suggestions made in the course of her calls she compiles a reasonably comprehensive list of the programs available in the community along with an idea of what they do and how much they cost. Her list includes a number of programs operated by hospital respiratory therapy departments as well as programs run by a variety of not-for-profit organizations.

Following this initial survey, Ms. Kelly begins Step 2, the evaluation of the service. She compiles a list of criteria which she considers essential in any program to which she will refer patients; the list is shown in Table 6.3. Ms. Kelly now contacts all of the programs which she feels may meet these criteria and asks the questions posed in Table 6.3. Seven programs, using a variety of techniques, appear to qualify. Typical is a program run by the American Cancer Society which offers a ten hour, week long "self help" program for $5.00, including free followup sessions.

Finally, Ms. Kelly schedules a visit to each of the qualifying programs to attend a typical session and obtain a better idea of what kind of patient will do best with the program's approach. She and a colleague will take about ten days to make the final evaluation and to make formal arrangements with the programs to accept her referrals (Step 3).

As a byproduct of her search Ms. Kelly discovers much free or low cost literature which her clinic can use. She believes some of this material may be helpful in dealing with patients who are not judged as candidates for a cessation program.

Table 6.3
A Checklist to Evaluate Smoking Cessation Programs.

1. How long has the program been operating?

   Criterion: The program should have been operating for at least one year unless special circumstances exist.

2. Is the program design based on the results of research and testing?

   Criterion: The approach used by the program should have some basis in research studies, preferably studies reported in a refereed journal.

3. Does the program have followup data which provide an estimate of the success of the program in promoting nonsmoking behavior? Does data indicate a reasonable success rate?

   Criterion: Data should exist which shows at least 30% nonsmoking behavior one year from participation. Claims of one year nonsmoking behavior of over 50% should be reviewed carefully for evidence of fraud.

4. Have the program instructors received formal training in how to conduct the program?

   Criterion: Program instructors should have received adequate training.

5. Is the program offered frequently enough so that patients can be referred without long delays?

   Criterion: Placement should be made within one month.

6. Is the program offered at reasonable cost to the patient?

   Criterion: For this example, cost must be under $30.00 per patient.

7. Is the program offered at a time and in a place acceptable to patients?

   Criterion: For this example, the time at which the program is offered is not considered important. (About half the patients work and would only be able to attend evening sessions; half do not, however, and could attend daytime sessions.) Place must be assessible by public transportation within one-half hour from the neighborhoods where the clinic draws its patients; travel should not be required in unsafe areas of the city.

From: Adapted from a checklist used by J. Fruetel, Mankato Health Promotion Program, Mankato, MN.

DEVELOPING INCOME FROM PREVENTIVE INITIATIVES

An important aspect of planning preventive initiatives is the way in which the practice recovers from the patients any costs which are associated with the provision of these initiatives, in particular:

- The cost associated with the time spent by the physicians involved with the patient's preventive care.

- The cost associated with the time spent by nonphysician practitioners in the practice who are involved with the patient's preventive care (nutritionist, counselor, nurse practitioner, and so forth).

- The cost associated with any expenses incurred on the patient's behalf (laboratory tests, patient education materials, and so forth).

- A reasonable allocation of the practice's overhead expenses (rent, heat, light, support personnel, and so forth).

In addition, the practice will want to consider the costs to the patient of services provided outside the practice used as an adjunct to the initiative sponsored by the practice. There are two important reasons for such planning:

- If the practice does not recover such costs from the patient (or from some third party) the practice will either become insolvent or will make up the costs by billing other services at a higher rate than necessary. When such overbilling occurs, it represents a subsidization of one service by another. Although not uncommon, such subsidization tends to distort the economics of practice and should be undertaken rarely and with caution.

- The cost to the patient of undertaking a preventive initiative may be an important factor in motivating the patient to participate in the initiative.

A key issue is the question of third-party coverage of the preventive initiatives provided by the practice. Most (about 90%) of Americans today have some kind of insurance against the costs associated with medical care; about 56% have insurance which covers outpatient care (for instance, care provided in the physician's office). Such outpatient care generally is associated with deductible and coinsurance limitations and is limited with respect to what is covered. As shown in Table 6.4 such limitations often exclude coverage of many preventive initiatives. However, experiments in preventive coverage exist.[6]

Most solo and group practice settings bill patients and third parties (on behalf of the patients) in all or part for the services which they provide (fee-for-service practice). Most hospital based clinics, neighborhood health centers, and the like also fall into this category.

Practice settings, such as HMOs and other institutions with responsibility for the patient's total health care on the basis of a flat premium payment or grant from the government, do not bill patients for services, preventive or otherwise, unless such services are somehow excluded from the "total" concept. For instance, many HMOs do not include dental care or drugs under their total care package; they often provide these services, however, and bill patients for them just as if they were a fee-for-service practice with respect to these services. Such organizations may or may not consider the provision of preventive initiatives to fall within their mandate.

Table 6.4
Third Party Coverage of Services Provided in an Outpatient, Fee-for-Service Setting

THIRD PARTY COVERAGE	OUTPATIENT SERVICE				COVERAGE FOR PREVENTIVE* SERVICE IN OUTPATIENT SETTING			
	DEDUCTIBLE	COPAYMENT	CONTROL	Note a	Note b	Note c	Note d
Blue Cross/Blue Shield	Maybe	Usual	Usual	Contract	Usual	Usually not	Usually not	Yes
Commerical	Maybe	Usual	Usual	Contract	Usual	Usually not	Usually not	Yes
Medicare (Part B)	Yes	Yes	Yes	Federal government	Yes	No	No	No
Medicaid	Yes	No	No	State/federal government	Yes	No	No	No †

* Assuming that outpatient coverage is offered.
† With the possible exception of some children's programs.
Note a. Covers diagnosis and treatment of recognized disease even though the thrust of the treatment is preventive. (Examples: high blood pressure, hyperlipidemia.)
Note b. Covers examination to discover aymptomatic disease with negative outcome. (Examples: Pap smear with negative outcome, mammogram with negative outcome.)
Note c. Covers health education and behavior modification to reduce risk.
Note d. Sponsors experimental progorams to test the coverage of preventive services of all types (notes a through c).

The decision by an HMO to include preventive initiatives is not made on the basis of ideal policy. Many of the considerations which are faced by a fee-for-service practice must be faced by an HMO as well. HMOs must compete with conventional insurance coverage schemes on the basis of the premium charged. Thus an HMO which takes on substantial commitments for preventive care may price itself out of the market when comparisons are made with an insurance company which has not elected to provide such coverage. Similar issues arise with government programs which underwrite health care for a particular group. The expenses to be incurred by including preventive initiatives in the care provided by the program can be accommodated only within certain budget constraints. These constraints often are established outside the control of the policy maker.

Thus, although the content of this section is most obviously applicable to fee-for-service practice, the cost issue raised must be considered by other types of practice in the process of policy making for the preventive initiatives.

To identify the cost and risk of introducing a preventive initiative, the following steps should be taken.

Step 1. __Estimate the first year's cost per patient to provide the preventive initiative.__ First estimate the cost to the practice, for the first year, to provide each new initiative for each patient who uses the initiative. You'll have to have a general idea of how the initiative is to be organized in order to do this; the development of a protocol and decisions on how to staff and what community resources to use should provide you with the necessary information.

- First consider the physician time in hours required over the first year for each patient in the initiative. For the moment don't worry where the time will come from. (If there is a solo practitioner who doesn't have the time available you may need to consider a part- or full-time associate to help with the initiative.) To associate a cost with this time, consider physician salary reduced to an hourly rate; if the physicians in the practice are not salaried pick a rate which you feel would adequately compensate for the time. Multiply the number of hours times the hourly rate to calculate cost.

- Second consider the time in hours required for each patient in the initiative over the first year from nonphysician personnel who will be involved with the initiative (nurse practitioner, psychologist, nutritionist, counselor, and so forth). To associate a cost with this time, consider the salary of such personnel reduced to an hourly rate. Multiply the number of hours times the hourly rate to calculate cost.

- Third consider the cost per patient associated with the initiative such as laboratory tests or educational materials paid for by the practice (not tests for which the patient will pay directly) over the first year of the initiative.

- Fourth allocate some of the practice's overhead cost (cost for heat, light, rent, telephone, support personnel, and so forth).

The total of these four categories represents the minimum which the practice must recover from each patient if the initiative is to be self supporting; it thus represents the minimum price that the practice should charge the patient.

Step 2. __Estimate any additional expense outside the practice which the patient will incur by virtue of joining your preventive initiative.__ Such expenses include testing, outside professional service referrals, and other outside programs which will be billed to the patient directly rather than through the practice. This total, together with the total of Step 1, represents the minimum price the patient can expect to pay for the initiative. It's important to know this figure in estimating the number of patients who will participate.

Step 3. Estimate utilization of the preventive initiatives. Begin by estimating the "market" for these initiatives, that is the number of individuals served by the practice each year to which a given preventive initiative would apply. Sort the market by age, sex, and insurance coverage since these are often important determinants of use. (Note that patients without insurance coverage or covered by Medicaid are usually not in a position to use services which require payment by the patient.)

Of the total market for each initiative estimate the number of patients who will use the initiative during the first year. Some elements of such an estimate relate to obvious and accessible facts: For instance the number of Medicaid and self-pay patients who will use a preventive initiative which they must pay for themselves will be low; they can't afford it. You must use your judgment and whatever expert opinion you can muster to consider other elements in the process by which a patient may decide to use a preventive initiative. Consider at least the following factors:

- age
- sex
- the price to the patient for the initiative (Steps 2 and 3 above)
- patient's income (use the kind of insurance coverage as a proxy for income)
- the amount of promotion you plan for the new initiative

In the occasional case that an insurance coverage exists for a preventive initiative, recent research suggests that you will find high utilization. Use Table 6.4 as a guideline; it may be necessary and desirable to conduct further research by making inquiries directly to the third parties insuring the patients served by the practice.

Your estimate of the use of the initiative provides important information as to the size of staff and other commitments you must have in place for the first year; these commitments, in turn, determine the risk to the practice in offering the initiative.

Step 4. Review your analysis for risk and fairness. In developing an initiative you will be incurring some risk. Two possible outcomes can result in loss of income.

- So far all costs have been considered "variable costs"; that is, costs will be proportional to the number of patients served. Realistically, however, some part of this cost structure should be represented as a "fixed cost." You will make commitments to add staff and for other purposes. If patient use does not develop to produce income offsetting these costs, the practice will lose money.

- Your estimates of cost may be too low. Even if patient use does develop as planned, you may still lose money.

Review your estimates. Decide what kind of commitments (fixed costs) you must make for the year in order to meet the expected use (Step 4 above). Then do a "worst-case" analysis. Assume your cost may be somewhat higher than estimated in Step 2 above and that use will be somewhat lower then estimated in Step 3 above; calculate how much money the practice will lose. If the practice loses enough money to threaten its solvency, you must rethink the initiatives. Either you cannot afford to offer them or you must scale them down to the point that, under the worst case, the practice remains solvent.

Your analysis may identify a group of patients who will not take advantage of the preventive initiative because of the out-of-pocket expense which they cannot afford, even though the initiative could be of great benefit to them. You may wish to increase the price of the initiative to the patients who can afford it and offer some "scholarships" to members of this group. (Don't forget to consider the effect of the increased price on initiative use.) You may wish to find a community resource as an alternative to your initiative if one exists with provision for service to low income patients.

As an example of the process described above, consider the case of a practice planning to add a smoking cessation initiative.

Income Analysis of a Smoking Cessation Initiative

Dr. Peter Schmidt and his practice were introduced above. An educated guess is that the yearly patient base looks something like that presented in Table 6.5.

Although the population is somewhat skewed towards the elderly population and they still see many patients with arthritis, Dr. Schmidt and Ms. Doyle are not surprised to find a number of younger patients with problems other than arthritis. The population has developed in two ways: Patients who originally came with arthritic problems naturally came with other problems; further, they recommended the practice to individuals who did not have arthritis problems at all. In fact, the practice is beginning to serve patients who are children and grandchildren of older patients. Because the original practice included many inner city patients referred to Dr. Schmidt by local neighborhood health centers and hospital clinics, a surprisingly large number of patients receive Medicaid.

Table 6.5
Patient Base for Dr. Pater Schmidt's Practice
(The numbers represent the population of individuals who come to Dr. Schmidt in the course of the year should they have a medical problem or wish a checkup.)

COVERAGE	MALE			FEMALE		
	<21	21-64	>64	<21	21-64	>64
Blue Cross/ Blue Shield or commercial insurer*	20	150	0	30	200	0
Self insured	2	15	0	3	20	0
Medicare	0	0	200	0	0	300
Medicaid †	10	20	50	20	50	50

* Not including supplementary policies.
† Patients over 65 on Medicaid also use Medicare; the state pays the part B premium for such patients and also reimburses copayments and deductibles.

Step 1. Estimate the first year's cost per patient to provide the new preventive initiative. Dr. Schmidt has found a psychologist who is willing to organize smoking cessation groups for patients served by the practice who wish to stop smoking. He proposes to deal with groups of ten patients; each group will receive ten one-hour sessions. In addition each participant will receive one hour of individual counseling from the psychologist. Thus two hours of the psychologist's time are required for each patient.

Ms. Doyle estimates she will have to spend an hour with each patient for initial assessment and counseling. Dr. Schmidt feels that he will have to spend about one-half hour per patient in assessing the patient's progress through the initiative. Dr. Schmidt and the psychologist discuss the use of thiocyanate laboratory tests to verify the patient's statements about his smoking; they decide not to include the tests at this point. Thus no direct expense other than the labor of the physician, the nurse, and the psychologist is involved in the initiative.

Finally Dr. Schmidt takes the advice of his accountant and adds $20 per patient to the cost of the initiative as an overhead allocation.

Thus the cost of the initiative per patient for the first year can be calculated as shown in Table 6.6.

Table 6.6
Estimate of the Cost per Patient per Year for a Smoking Cessation Initiative

Physician: 1/2 hour @ $50/hour	$25
Nurse practitioner: 1 hour @ $30/hour	$30
Psychologist: 2 hours @ $35/hour	$70
Overhead allocation	$20
TOTAL	$145

Step 2. Estimate any additional expense outside the practice which the patient will incur by virtue of joining the preventive initiative. The only outside expenses which the patient must bear are casual costs associated with transportation to and from the sessions and appointments.

Step 3. Estimate use of the new preventive initiative. Dr. Schmidt decides to estimate the number of smokers among his patients on the basis of national statistics available from the federal government. He sends his secretary to the university library and she returns with the following information (Table 6.7.)

Table 6.7
Percentage of Smokers

	------- MALE -------			------- FEMALE -------		
	<21	21-64	>64	<21	21-64	>64
	30	70	50	35	50	25

From the information in Table 6.7 a market table can be constructed which gives some idea as to the number of patients who are potential users of the practice's smoking cessations initiative; the number in Table 6.5 is multiplied by the corresponding percentages in Table 6.7. The results are shown in Table 6.8.

Dr. Schmidt must now make the hardest part of the calculation, an estimate of the number of patients out of the market who will actually use his smoking cessation initiative during the first year. Dr. Schmidt uses Table 6.4 and consults with a few third parties (Blue Cross/Blue Shield, two of the largest commercial carriers in the area, the local intermediary for Medicare, and the state welfare office). He comes to the conclusion that little or no part of the smoking cessation initiative will be reimbursed by a third party.

Table 6.8
Market for Dr. Schmidt's Smoking Cessation Initiative

	------ MALE ------			------ FEMALE ------		
COVERAGE	<21	21-64	>64	<21	21-64	>64
Blue Cross/ Blue Shield or commercial insurer	6	105	0	11	100	0
Self insured	1	11	0	1	10	0
Medicare	0	0	100	0	0	75
Medicaid	3	14	25	7	25	13

Dr. Schmidt consults further with a counselor at the local branch of the American Lung Association who has experience with smoking cessation programs organized by the Association. He decides that he will attract 10% of his market except for self-insured patients and Medicaid patients; he assumes he will attract none of the self-insured or Medicaid patients if the minimum price must be $145.00. Table 6.9 results. He therefore predicts use by 41 patients during the first year.

Table 6.9
Projected Utilization of Dr. Schmidt's Smoking Cessation Initiative for the First Year

	------ MALE ------			------ FEMALE ------		
COVERAGE	<21	21-64	>64	<21	21-64	>64
Blue Cross/ Blue Shield or commercial insurer	1	11	0	1	10	0
Self insured	0	0	0	0	0	0
Medicare	0	0	10	0	0	8
Medicaid	0	0	0	0	0	0

Step 4. Review the analysis for risk and fairness. Dr. Schmidt finds that if he wants to have the capacity for 41 patients in place he must commit to using 100 hours of the psychologist's time in the coming year ($3,500) whether or not the patients take the initiative. Under very pessimistic assumptions, perhaps only 25 patients would actually join the initiative and he and Ms. Doyle might have to spend more time per patient than anticipated. Even though he and Ms. Doyle can adjust their time to the actual patient load, and assuming the price of the initiative will be $145.00 per patient, the practice would be exposed to a loss in the worst case:

```
Income:  25 patients x $145/patient...............$3,625
Expense: physician: 25 patients x $50/patient....(1,250)
         nurse practitioner: 25 patients x $45/
                             patient..............(1,125)
         psychologist............................(3,500)
         overhead: 25 patients x $20/patient.......(500)
                                                 --------
(Loss)..........................................($2,750)
```

Dr. Schmidt views this as an acceptable risk to the practice and decides to proceed. He and Ms. Doyle are concerned about their population of self-insured and Medicaid patients. They know that they need the initiative just as much as his more well to do patients. On the other hand, they don't want to discourage participation by pricing the initiative at more than $145 per patient until they have some experience. Ms. Doyle decides to investigate community resources for programs to which they might refer patients who are unable to afford the practice's initiative. Next year it may be possible to adjust the pricing so that a few scholarships can be offered.

INFORMATION SYSTEMS

Ideally information about a patient's experience in a preventive initiative would be integrated with information on other preventive initiatives which the practice provides for the patient. Information on which risks a patient faces is often collected as a part of an initial health and risk assessment (see Chapter 3), for which many different instruments exist. The information provided from such assessments forms a base line for the patient: for instance, does he smoke? What is his blood pressure? Is cholesterol level a problem? Once the baseline data is collected, however, each practice may use different intervention strategies and will need to develop appropriate information systems.

Information systems used to support preventive initiatives are different than some traditionally used to support acute medical care intervention. Among the special characteristics of an information system developed for a preventive initiative are accommodation of a recurring stream of assessment and intervention data and accommodation of information which can be used to evaluate the initiative.

As a procedure for developing an information system, take the following steps for each preventive initiative implemented by the practice:

Step 1. Develop objectives for the information system. Review the protocol for the preventive initiative you wish to implement. Specify what information should be made available in the form of reports, to whom and when it should be supplied, and what action should result from the information.

Step 2. Specify information input. Identify the information which must be collected in order to meet the objectives developed in step 1.

Reference to the flow chart describing the protocol is helpful in identifying the points at which information must be collected and identifying the person who is to collect it.

Design any forms required to facilitate the recording of the information.

Step 3. Design a record to contain the information. At this point we need a single, central depository for all of the information being collected. This depository is usually most easily arranged on the basis of a record for each patient in the preventive initiative. As the next section indicates, it is helpful to design the record so that the information it contains can be entered in a computer.

Step 4. Design procedures for processing the records to provide the reports identified in step 1. The final step in implementing an information system is to develop the procedures necessary to read the records prepared as a result of the design of Step 3 and, using this information, to prepare the reports identified in Step 1. As a part of this process, the person responsible for the preparation of reports should be identified. The process may be carried out manually or by machine; if a machine is to be used, the procedure will include the preparation of any computer programs necessary to read the records and prepare reports as discussed in the next section.

An Information System for a Smoking Cessation Initiative

In the following material the flow chart of Figure 6.1 is assumed to describe the protocol for the preventive initiative. Material in quotation marks refers to the titles of the activity and decision boxes in the flow chart.

Step 1. Develop objectives for the information system. Reviewing the protocol in Figure 6.1 the following reports would seem desirable.

REPORT	TO WHOM	WHEN
Patient's smoking history	Person performing "assess by interview"	At interview
Patient scheduled for reassessment	Person responsible for "patient still accessible to practice"	One month prior to scheduled reassessment
Cessation program evaluation	Person responsible for preventive initiative management	Yearly

Step 2. Specify information input. The first piece of information required is the date of the history and an indica-

tion of whether the patient smokes at that time. The individual taking the history provides this information. The history may be a health risk assessment.

The person responsible for the two subsequent steps for patients identified as smokers "assess by interview" and "candidate for cessation program?" must provide information as to whether the patient has been referred to a cessation program (either in house or through the use of a community resource).

The person responsible for "assessing program result" or the person responsible for "counsel" must supply the suggested time for the next assessment. In addition, if the patient has been referred to a cessation program, the person responsible for "assess program result" must provide information on the putative result of the program.

All of these information inputs will become a part of the patient's record (see Step 3). Since the inputs come from different people at different times, some thought must be given to how the information gets to the individual responsible for maintaining the record. Simple forms may be designed to allow each individual responsible for information input to provide the data to the individual responsible for maintaining the record.

Step 3. Design a record to contain the information input. All of the above information input can be contained in a single record, based on the patient (Figure 6.3). The record is initiated at the time of the first history and may be maintained in written form by an appropriate responsible individual, as indicated in Step 2 above.

The same record may be maintained in a computer by the individual responsible for maintaining the record. If reasonable backup of computer records is practiced, a separate, written record is not necessary. Although making the computer entries will save no time over making manual entries, the process of producing reports will be greatly speeded.

In the example shown in Figure 6.3, patient Wolfgang A. Mozart has a history first taken October 10, 1980, at which time he admits to smoking three packs of cigarettes a day. Following assessment, he is assigned to smoking cessation program number 3; the assessment which follows the cessation program results in a pessimistic prognosis (value 2) and assigns reassessment at a year from his first appointment.

At this time he is still accessible to the practice and enters cycle two of the program on December 3, 1981. Sure enough, he is still a three-pack-a-day man. At assessment, the decision is made not to try another cessation program

PATIENT NAME: <u>MOZART   WOLFGAN A</u>
                     1   15 16   23 24

ADDRESS: <u>52 LOUDER'S LANE</u>
              25   49
<u>BOSTON</u>
50   67
<u>MA 02130</u>
68   74

CYCLE	A	B	C	D	E	F
1	<u>80101 0</u>	<u>9</u>	<u>3</u>	<u>2</u>	<u>8/0/10</u>	<u>A</u>
	75	80	81	82	83 84	89 90
2	<u>81203</u>	<u>9</u>	<u>0</u>	<u>4</u>	<u>82/203</u>	<u>A</u>
	91	96	97	98	99 100	101 102
3	<u>82/130</u>	<u>0</u>	<u>0</u>	<u>9</u>	<u>841130</u>	
	103	108	109	110	111 112	113 114

(etc.)

<u>Figure 6.3.</u> Patient record for protocol shown in Figure 6.1. Ten cycles or more through the protocol can easily fit on a single page, covering a time period ranging from 10 to 50 years, depending on the frequency of reassessment. The numbers below the lines indicate the spaces reserved in a computer record for the information; ten cycles would require about 200 character spaces reserved; using a small (5-1/4 inch) disk of the "double-density" type, about 1,500 records could be placed on a single disk.

Column A contains the date of the first and subsequent history/ assessments. Column B contains a number rating the severity of smoking behavior as determined at the time of the history assessment; 0 is a nonsmoker, 9 is over three packs a day. Column C contains a number indicating which smoking cessation program the patient was referred to; 0 indicates no referral (counseling option). Column D provides a rating from 0 to 9 of the prognosis following the cessation program; 0 indicates no change likely, 9 indicates high likelihood of complete cessation. Column E is the date for next assessment assigned by the individual evaluating the result of the cessation program or providing the counseling (or, in the case of a nonsmoker, the history taker, who assigns a date on the basis of the reassessment times recommended.) Column F is filled in at the time an attempt is made to recontact the patient for his next assessment; A indicates the patient is accessible to the practice, N that he is not.

(0 indication in column C); instead Mr. Mozart is counseled. The counselor is hopeful following their session and assigns a value of 4 to the prognosis. The counselor still wants to see Mozart again in a year. Mozart is still accessible to the practice at that time (cycle 3) and, mirabile dictu, he's stopped smoking. At this point the history taker assigns him for reassessment two years hence.

Step 4. Design programs for processing the records to provide the reports identified in Step 1. In a manual system, each record would be filed alphabetically. At the time a reassessment date is assigned, a separate 3"x5" card with the patient's name and reassessment date is filed in a "tickler" file arranged by month over a five year period. Thus in the month prior to the tickler entry, the person responsible for "patient still accessible to practice?" can attempt to contact all patients scheduled for reassessment in the next month and set up appointments for reassessment. (If the reassessments deals only with smoking, the process does not require the patient to come in if the patient simply states he does not smoke.)

In this case, the tickler file represents the necessary report.

In a manual system the second report requirement can be met by simply providing the patient record to the person responsible for assessment and the person responsible for counseling or running the cessation program.

The evaluation of cessation program success is the most difficult to generate using a manual system. One would have to sort through the alphabetically filed record forms to find individuals who had been through the program in question and tabulate the results as reported at the "assess program result" point in the protocol. If reassessment information is available subsequent to the cessation program, it would be useful to know if the patient is or is not smoking at the time he is reassessed.

Unsophisticated computer programs may be used to generate these reports if the records have been placed in a computer file. The most simple approach is to have the computer read every record in the file to extract whatever information is desired. It may seem wasteful to ask the computer to read every record (there may be thousands) to identify a group of patients whose reassessment is coming due (there may be only a handful). However, because the machine can work with blind, mindless speed, the method is reasonable.

The next section will amplify some of the other advantages of computer use. For instance: the computer can print address labels for patients due for reassessment (for reminders); the computer can write a much more readable report than provided in Figure 6.3.

USING COMPUTERS TO MANAGE A PREVENTIVE INITIATIVE

Computers can be useful in the management of preventive initiatives. Until recently, only a large group practice or an institutional practice could consider the use of a computer. Within the past few years, however, very sophisticated, low cost machines have become available. Today even the smallest practice can afford such equipment; so called "personal computers" with printer and software cost no more than $2,000-3,000. This equipment has the power of computers which, not more than a few years ago, would have been completely outside the means of all but the largest practices.

A potential user of a personal computer must choose between machines which run the PC/DOS or MS/DOS operating system[8] (for instance IBM[9] and IBM compatible[10] machines) and those which use other operating systems (for instance Apple[11] machines). It is likely that any computer programs which you may wish to use will be available in some form for either operating system, although they are more likely to be available first for the /DOS operating system.

Literally hundreds of programs are available for performing routine practice management tasks: word processing (letter writing) and accounting programs for instance. A few practices are experimenting with more specialized programs designed for the field of prevention[12], including programs which produce health risk assessments. For the routine record-keeping tasks described in the last section, a number of "data base" programs are available.

As an example of how a data base program is used, the Ashton-Tate product dBase[13] may be applied to the form illustrated in Figure 6.3. This program allows the user to create an electronic record analogous to the paper record shown in the figure. The process proceeds in two steps:

- In Step 1, the user creates a record format which has the same format as the paper record. The process identifies the various blocks of information ("fields") on the form as to length and whether they contain numerical or textual information. Each field is assigned a name by which it can be accessed.

- In Step 2, the user creates a record for each patient in the program. The dBase program asks the user to type in the relevant information for each field for each patient; it then assigns a number to each patient record and stores the records permanently on a magnetic disk. Records can be added, removed, or changed at any time.

The dBase program can be used to access the file of patient records for various purposes. For instance, the program can search the file for patients due for reassessment, thereby supplanting the tickler file described in the previous section. The program can print mailing labels for these patients. The program will search the file for patient Mozart and will print out his record, thereby providing a written record which will be available when Mozart comes in for reassessment. This record can be formatted in a much more readable form than shown in Figure 6.3. The program can tabulate the assessment of program results for each intervention offered by the practice to provide evaluation results. Thus the dBase program can support all of the requirements of the information system described in the example of the last section.

The use of a machine to support an information system must be justified on the basis of the saving of clerical and professional time and the elimination of costly errors which are implicit in the use of the machine. These savings must be set against the cost of the machine and the not inconsiderable time and trouble to train the staff in its use and to properly maintain the records.

The cost saving tends to recur with time and to increase as the number of records increases; the cost tends to be a front-end cost, the amount of which is independent of the number of records. Thus there is generally a number of records at which machine processing becomes effective. The front-end cost is low enough, however, so that even a small practice is likely to generate enough records to justify the use of a machine, particularly if the information system can be supported by an existing applications program such as dBase.

REFERENCES

1. Awad EM: <u>Business Data Processing</u>, ed 4. Englewood Cliffs (New Jersey), Prentice-Hall, Inc., 1975.

2. Lewy R: <u>Preventive Primary Medicine</u>. Boston, Little, Brown and Co., 1980.

3. Rund D: Problem solving. In Taylor RB et al (eds): <u>Family Medicine: Principles and Practice.</u> New York, Springer Verlag, 1978.

4. DeAngelis C: Non-physician health care providers and community support services. <u>Pediatric Clinics of North America</u> 28:551-563, 1981.

5. Pender NJ and Pender AR: Illness prevention and health promotion services provided by nurse practitioners: predicting potential consumers. <u>AJPH</u> 70:798-804, 1980.

6. Mauksch IG: Nurse-physician collaboration: a changing relationship. <u>Journal of Nursing Administration</u> 11(6):35-38, 1981.

7. The Insure Project on Lifecycle Preventive Health Services Project, 330 Park Ave. South, New York, NY 10010.

8. The PC/DOS and MS/DOS operating systems are products of Microsoft Corporation, Bellevue, Washington 98004.

9. IBM Corporation, Entry Systems Division, 1000 NW 51st St., Boca Raton, Florida 33432.

10. There are many manufacturers of IBM compatible equipment, e.g.:
    Compaq Computer, Houston, Texas.
    AT&T Information Systems, Iselin, New Jersey 08830.
    Leading Edge Hardware Products, Inc., 225 Turnpike St., Canton, Massachusetts 02021.

11. Apple Computer, 20525 Mariani Ave., Cupertino, California 95014.

12. Hattwick MA et al: Using the information tool to improve preventive medical care. In Proceedings of the Fifth Annual Symposium on Computer Care. McLean (Virginia), Medical Information Management, Inc., 1981.

13. Ashton-Tate, 10150 West Jefferson Boulevard, Culver City, California 90230.

CHAPTER 7

The Cinderella Effect: Good Teaching Will Transform the Practice of Preventive Medicine

Hannelore F. Vanderschmidt, Ph.D.

THE PROBLEM

Enlightened teaching in preventive medicine is bound to produce a "Cinderella effect." From grubby housemaid, cleaning the ashes from the fireplace, doing the jobs nobody wants to do, we intend to elevate her to the status of beautiful maiden wooed by Prince Charming, turned out in a fashionable gown and slippers and transported by a golden coach.

In a nation where half of the deaths are preventable,[1] where cigarette smoking alone is responsible for 485,000 deaths per year,[2] faculties are still only paying lip service to the training of health professionals, including physicians and nurses, in skills associated with the clinical prevention of disease.

Courses dealing with preventive medicine comprise only 1.5% of medical school courses.[3] In nursing the picture is similar. Prevention broadly defined is emphasized but still constitutes only a small fraction of the curriculum.

Not only are courses in prevention few, but they are poorly taught, often relying on standard texts and didactic teaching. Only rarely do they give students access to a clinical site or let them see their role models (doctors, nurses, and other providers) practicing preventive medicine as it is presently conceived. (See Chapter 3—The Methods of Clinical Health Maintenance.) When courses are perceived to be irrelevant and dull, graduates will have little incentive to remember course content or to utilize course related concepts in their professional practice.

Derek Bok, President of Harvard University, decries the quality and the quantity of preventive medicine teaching in the U.S.:

> To begin with, faculties can offer better instruction in preventive medicine. Up to half of all illness in the United States could be avoided through changes in behavior brought about by voluntary adjustments in lifestyle or by preventive measures on the part of government and private organizations. The latter are primarily the responsibility of the

state acting through appropriate rules and incentives. But education and persuasion can bring individuals to avoid smoking, excessive drinking, dietary deficiencies, inadequate exercise, unknowing exposure to health hazards, and many other forms of dangerous behavior. In this endeavor, the media and the schools have important roles to play. But physicians have a special competence to discover risks that patients unwittingly run in their daily lives. They also have a special status and authority that can help them persuade individuals to alter their habits. Yet prevention currently receives only 1.5 percent of total teaching time in the medical curriculum. One should not exaggerate the impact of more instruction-- we know too little about the process of changing human behavior. Even so, there is little doubt that doctors could learn to be more effective in detecting avoidable causes of disease, more competent in using epidemiological techniques to identify community measures for prevention, and more adept at persuading patients to minimize needless risks. With greater numbers of primary care practitioners and the growth of health maintenance organizations and other community-based institutions for health care, the opportunities for doctors to make such contributions seem destined to increase.[3]

For those who have graduated from medical and nursing schools, there is a paucity of continuing education courses in prevention. It is only in the last ten years that preventive protocols have been clearly defined and that clinical prevention has developed a substantial research base. Providers who were students more than ten years ago may never have studied clinical prevention or perceived that their health maintenance skills are limited. In a performance analysis of physicians and nursing competencies in clinical prevention carried out by the Center for Educational Development in Health/Association of Teachers of Preventive Medicine, we found that practicing physicians and nurses agreed that their skills in implementing clinical health maintenance programs, especially their skill in helping patients to modify their lifestyle, were insufficient.[4] Another recent study substantiates this point.[5] Over 80% of a sample of 1,040 practicing primary care physicians reported that their skills in modifying patient behavior was insufficient. When a health professions work force recognizes its own insufficiency with respect to prevention, high quality continuing education courses are a high priority.

Finally, competency based approaches to designing curriculum in the preventive domain are seldom applied. Competency based courses look at the job health professionals perform at the work place in order to derive objectives and content for instruction. Competency based training techniques have been used to structure some medical/nursing education in the United States, and techniques for developing such courses are available. Yet very few prevention oriented courses apply the techniques. For example, questions such as the following are seldom asked: What should the practicing doctor, nurse, nutritionist, health educator, know about the smoking risk? What skills are needed to confront smoking patients? How does one implement a smoking cessation program? How does the provider evaluate the effectiveness of such a course of treatment? How long does he/she follow up and how?

ASSUMPTIONS

It is assumed that most health professionals do some teaching in formal courses or seminars and in informal, often impromptu, 'how to do it' sessions involving colleagues or employees. It is assumed further that good teaching in preventive medicine has a clinical component and that training physicians, nurses, and other members of the health team includes aspects of both vertical and horizontal integration.

In vertical (topdown) integration (Figure 7.1) residents and graduate nurses learn to deliver preventive skills in a clinical site: office, HMO, clinic, etc. and they in turn become role models for third and fourth year students who have a preventive medicine clerkship/rotation at a clinical site. First and second year courses are structured to provide the necessary knowledge and skills to enable the student to work under supervision in the subsequent clinical rotation. Preventive initiatives need not be taught in courses in prevention per se. Integration into courses such as pediatrics, gerontology, cardiovascular disease, infectious/communicable disease, malignant neoplasms, etc. is encouraged.

It is further assumed that members of the health team (doctors, nurses, psychologists, nutritionists) work as a team in providing preventive services. Since the team approach seems the only realistic one in providing such a complex range of services, it follows that medical and nursing students would do well to study together both in the class and the practicum setting. Such an integrated approach is here called horizontal integration (Figure 7.2).

GOALS AND OBJECTIVES

The ultimate goals of teaching clinical prevention are to:

- optimize the quality of preventive services;
- provide a range of services to a large and diverse client population;
- enable health providers to develop new and better preventive services as they have developed innovations in curative medicine.

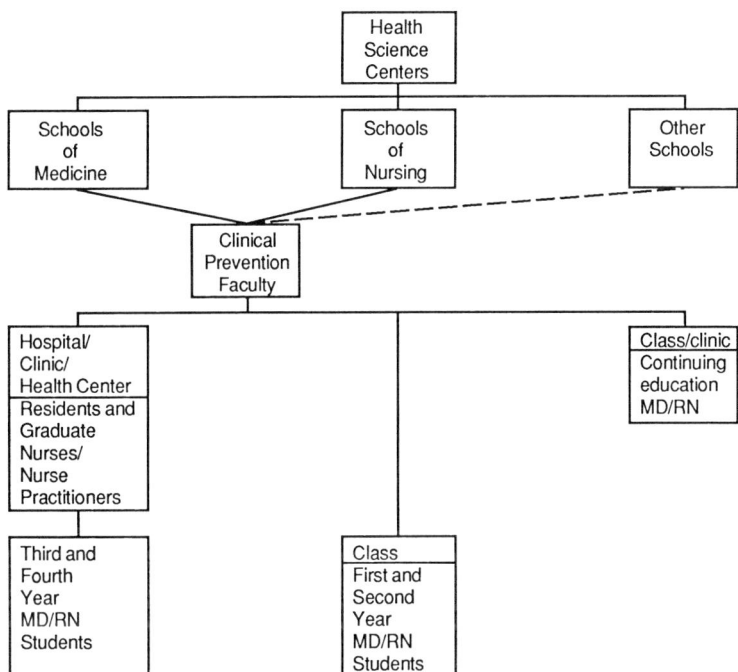

Figure 7.1. Education of physicians and nurses in clinical prevention using a 'top-down' approach. Health science centers utilize providers working at clinical sites as faculty for residents as well as CME/Continuing Education workshops. In turn, residents teach undergraduate medical and nursing students in clinical clerkships/practice at the clinical sites. First and second year students are taught the knowledge of clinical prevention by clinicians and other faculty members.

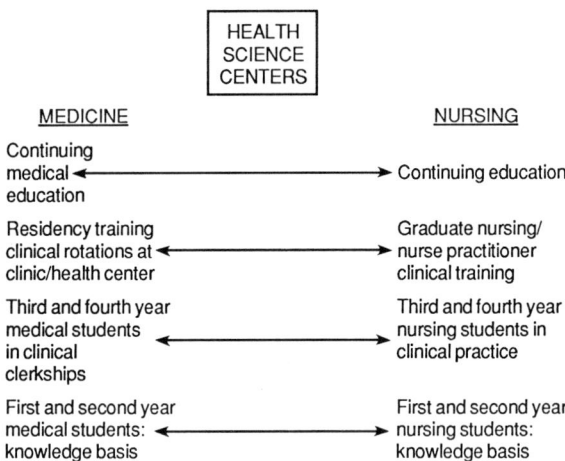

Figure 7.2. Health science centers showing horizontal integration in clinical prevention. Residency training and training of graduate nurses is accomplished at a clinical site with both medical and nursing providers working together. Residents/graduate nurses in turn teach third and fourth year medical/nursing students in clinical clerkships/practica. Finally, first and second year nursing and medical students learn the concepotual framework of clinical prevention in close coordination with the clinical requirements.

The specific objectives include developing skills, knowledge and attitude with respect to health promotion and disease prevention. These include the ability to:

- discuss health promotion initiatives—risk, primary and secondary prevention of disease;
- interpret recent epidemiologic studies concerning prevention of disease;
- describe the main areas of risk where preventive interventions are presently available;
- plan and manage preventive components of practice;
- implement clinical health maintenance procedures including risk assessment, planning, implementing, and evaluating health maintenance programs.

(See the ATPM objectives in health promotion and disease prevention.[6])

TARGET POPULATION

Since clinical preventive medicine requires such a range and complexity of competencies, a mix of professions should be involved as students, teachers, and providers. Nurses, doctors, social workers, nutritionists, health educators and psychologists should be included in the preventive health care team.

PLANNING COURSES

Courses and entire curricula for health professional teaching programs should be derived from the tasks which individuals are expected to carry out on the job. By focusing on the job, rather than on a long list of concepts, theories and memorized procedures which have traditionally been part of an instructional program, the teacher enables the student to become an effective worker after leaving school.

Although competency based approaches focus on performance, they require the student to acquire background theory and knowledge so that performance is informed, not merely mechanical. Competency based training approaches also call for development of positive attitudes towards the patient and towards provision of services.[7]

Using the competency based training methods we suggest that teachers planning their course develop objectives for instruction in behavioral terms and that these objectives be based on the necessary job skills, knowledge and attitudes (Table 7.1).

Table 7.1
Outline of Instructional Unit on Designing Patient Flow Patterns

		OBJECTIVE		HOURS	
	SESSION TITLE	GIVEN	STUDENT WILL	CL	PR
0.	Entry level	A description of a simple process such as billing	Design a flow chart describing the process using branches and loops as necessary.	NA	NA
1.	Review of a preventive initiative	A description of a practice population	Summarize the application of a health promotion initiative (such as a physical fitness program) or a disease prevention program (such as smoking cessation or hypertension control) to the population.	0	3
2.	Charting patient flow in a preventive program	A description of a practice setting	Produce a flow diagram with branches and loops as necessary for a preventive initiative undertaken by the practice.	1	3
			TOTAL	1	6

Having developed objectives, instructional activities should be planned to enable students to acquire the skills included in each objective. Activities listed in Example 7.1 might be included in teaching objective 2. (See also the flow chart in Figure 6.1.)

When students become involved in the instructional process, they develop skills and attitudes. Didactic teaching may require less preparation on the part of the teacher but it often results in individuals with a low skill level and a lack of interest in the subject—a person who remembers facts and definitions but is only marginally able to apply these to solve problems. Learning activities where the students become actively involved include case discussions, exercises, patient management problems—projects where students have an opportunity to practice prevention related skills in a real or simulated setting.

Example 7:1
Sample Session Plan

SESSION 2: CHARTING PATIENT FLOW IN A PREVENTIVE PROGRAM

Objective of Session 2

Given a description of a practice setting the student will produce a flow diagram with branches and loops as necessary for a preventive initiative undertaken by the practice.

Reading for Session 2

Benfari RC: Lifestyle alteration and the primary prevention of CHD: the Multiple Risk Factor Intervention Trial (MRFIT). Intervention Sudies, 341-351.

The article describes the protocol used in the MRFIT program which attempted to control smoking, hypertension and diet for a group of individuals at high risk for coronary heart disease over the course of over five years.

Student Activity for Session 2

Assign one of the practice settings from the Learning Resources volume for Module II to each of the students. Ask each student to prepare a flow chart showing a protocol for dealing with the patients in this practice for whichever of the preventive initiatives you decide to use (see Session 1).

When you receive the flow charts, pick one example from each practice setting, and put the chart on a viewgraph transparency. Schedule a class and ask the student responsible for each of the charts which you picked to explain the flow chart to the rest of the class. Open the floor to discussion following each presentation. Lead the discussion to bring out the most significant aspects of the way in which patients access services and the way in which assessment and intervention are sequenced.

Your students' flow charts should resemble Figure 6-1.

EVALUATION

In designing a training program on clinical prevention, the instructor will want to test students to determine if they have mastered the critical skills as identified in the objectives of the course.

Determination of which sort of testing method to choose is made by analyzing the skills which are to be evaluated. Clinical skills such as taking a preventive history or counseling patients with respect to risk reduction are best evaluated by organizing a real or simulated situation where the student does the workup. A checklist is developed by the instructor to determine if the student asks the important questions, probes, and asks for clarification as needed. Ability to interpret a risk assessment questionnaire (or a computerized health risk assessment) and to communicate results to the patient can be tested in a similar fashion. (See Chapter 3 for an example of a risk assessment questionnaire.)

In each case the instructor needs to develop the scenario or simulated case materials and a checklist of critical answers by which to evaluate the student. Tables 7.2 and 7.3. illustrate two performance checklists.

The advantage of a performance testing mechanism is that it has face validity: The student is being tested in procedures and circumstances that are identical to the conditions in the office or clinic. Performance tests, however, are time consuming to administer since each student must be evaluated separately. Teaching assistants may be taught to administer performance tests, so as to lighten instructor workload. In this case, instructors must give clear, written instructions as well as the checklists and score keys to teaching assistants to assure that every student is evaluated the same way.

Objectives and checklists can be shared with students at the beginning of the course so that the student will be able to practice to perfection on similar problems. Of course, the students may not consult the checklist during testing. In this way the students are apprised of the competencies which they will be asked to demonstrate at the end of the course.

In an epidemiology course the instructor may wish to ask students to analyze a journal article or to solve representative problems. Objective, multiple choice, short answer tests are valuable in testing the knowledge basis. While these tests are easy to score, it is difficult to write items which require high level analytic or problem solving skills.

Student attitudes are probably best gauged through anonymous questionnaires. Students usually know the right answer to a test of attitude. Anonymity will provide more honest responses. An example of a questionnaire to gauge attitudes with respect to preventive medicine teaching is shown in Table 7.4.

Table 7.2
Clinical Evaluation Guide

This checklist outlines critical points of performance in the planning and implementation of health maintenance/health promotion services as part of community health nursing. It is intended for use in evaluating the skills of students during their education and practice of nursing in the community.

PLAN   COMMENTS

1. Bases plan of care on assessment data.
2. Obtains input from community agencies involved with client.
3. Plans with the client to meet health needs.
4. Uses contracting process in interactions with clients to encourage self care.
5. Prepares appropriate care plan on each family in caseload.

IMPLEMENTATION

1. Delivers planned nursing services.
2. Directs care to secondary and tertiary levels of prevention, with anticipatory guidance directed toward primary prevention.
3. Recognizes changing focus of client's needs; promptly adapts plan of care to respond to new needs.
4. Serves all families in caseload through effective case management.
5. Utilizes appropriate community resources.
6. Collaborates with other members of the health team; maintains open communication with appropriate personnel.
7. Observes and begins to perform Community Health Nursing skills in the clinic setting designed to meet specific health needs of a client group.
8. Teaches a health related topic to a group of adolescents.

From: Herman M: Clinical Evaluation Guide (excerpt). Loma Linda, CA: Loma Linda University, School of Nursing, 1985. Reprinted by permission.

Table 7.3
Example of a Performance Checklist.

This checklist assesses competencies in data gathering, recording, and interpreting, in the performance of a cardiovascular examination. Emphasis is placed on the ability to perform according to specific actions and to conduct a thorough examination. The purpose of this assessment is summative.

CARDIOVASCULAR EXAMINATION PERFORMANCE CHECK-LIST

Examiner's name _____ Patient's name _____ Date _____

A. *General inspection/ vital signs*
- ____ 1. Wash hands before starting examination.
- ____ 2. Measure blood pressure in right upper limb, sitting or lying.
- ____ 3. Measure blood pressure in left upper limb, sitting or lying.
- ____ 4. Measure blood pressure in either upper limb, standing.
- ____ 5. Empty cuff completely before inflating it.
- ____ 6. Measure respiratory rate for at least 60 seconds.
- ____ 7. Palpate radial pulse for at least 15 seconds.
- ____ 8. Palpate radial pulse simultaneously for symmetry.

B. *Hands and arms*
- ____ 1. Inspect both hands.

C. *Head and neck*
- ____ 1. Palpate carotids bilaterally.
- ____ 2. Auscultate carotids bilaterally.

D. *Lungs*
- ____ 1. Ask patient to cross arms to move scapulae and expose lung fields.
- ____ 2. Percuss posterior lung fields.
- ____ 3. Percuss fields bilaterally and symmetrically, in all areas.
- ____ 4. Instruct patient to breathe through open mouth.
- ____ 5. Auscultate posterior lung fields.
- ____ 6. Auscultate all areas bilaterally and symmetrically with patient breathing through open mouth.

Lateral lung fields
- ____ 7. Percuss lateral lung fields
- ____ 8. Auscultate lateral lung fields.

Anterior lung fields
- ____ 9. Percuss anterior lung fields.
- ____ 10. Percuss fields bilaterally and symmetrically.
- ____ 11. Auscultate anterior lung fields.
- ____ 12. Auscultate anterior lung fields bilaterally and symmetrically.

E. *Heart*
- ____ 1. Observe precordium.

Palpate with patient *sitting*:
- ____ 2. Aortic area (2nd ICS - right).
- ____ 3. Pulmonic area (2nd and 3rd ICS - left).
- ____ 4. Right ventricular area.
- ____ 5. Apical area (5th ICS - left)

Auscultate with patient *sitting* (using diaphragm of stethoscope):
- ____ 6. Aortic area.
- ____ 7. Pulmonic area.
- ____ 8. Tricuspid area (4th and 5th ICS at left sternal edge).
- ____ 9. Mitral (apical) area.

Auscultate with patient *sitting* (using *bell* of stethoscope):
- ____ 10. Aortic area.
- ____ 11. Pulmonic area.
- ____ 12. Tricuspid area.
- ____ 13. Apical area.
- ____ 14. *Observe* neck veins with patient in *recumbent* position.

Palpate with patient *recumbent*:
- ____ 15. Aortic area (2nd ICS - right).
- ____ 16. Pulmonic area (2nd and 3rd ICS - left).
- ____ 17. Right ventricular area.
- ____ 18. Apical area (5th ICS - left).
- ____ 19. Ectopic area (between right ventricular and apical areas)

From: Katz FM and Snow R: Assessing Health Workers' Performance: A Manual for Training and Supervision. Geneva, Switzerland: World Health Organization, 1980, p. 135.

Table 7.3 (Cont'd.)
Example of a Performance Checklist.

Auscultate with patient *recumbent* (using diaphragm of stethoscope):
- _____ 20. Aortic area.
- _____ 21. Pulmonic area.
- _____ 22. Tricuspid area
- _____ 23. Mitral (apical) area.

Auscultate with patient *recumbent* (using *bell* of stethoscope):
- _____ 24. Aortic area.
- _____ 25. Pulmonic area.
- _____ 26. Tricuspid area.
- _____ 27. Mitral area.
- _____ 28. Ask patient to roll to left lateral position.
- _____ 29. Relocate apex.
- _____ 30. Auscultate apex with bell.
- _____ 31. Auscultate apex with diaphragm.

F. Abdomen
- _____ 1. Patient is taught to relax abdominal musculature.
- _____ 2. Watch patient's face as you examine abdomen.
- _____ 3. Auscultate before manipulation or palpation.

Auscultate
- _____ 4. Aorta.
- _____ 5. Renal arteries.
- _____ 6. Iliac arteries.
- _____ 7. Palpate epigastrium superficially.
- _____ 8. Palpate epigastrium deeply.
- _____ 9. Palpate right upper quadrant.
- _____ 10. Use proper technique to palpate liver edge.
- _____ 11. Percuss liver span.
- _____ 12. Palpate left upper quadrant.
- _____ 13. Use proper technique to palpate tip of spleen.

G. Lower limbs
- _____ 1. Inspect bilaterally with outer clothes removed.
- _____ 2. Inspect feet including toes

Palpate pulses bilaterally:
- _____ 3. Femoral
- _____ 4. Popliteal.
- _____ 5. Posterior tibial.
- _____ 6. Dorsalis pedis.
- _____ 7. Auscultate for femoral bruits.
- _____ 8. Check for peripheral pitting edema
- _____ 9. Use proper technique to check for pitting edema.

Total score obtained _____ Total score possible 76

For the evaluator Key: 5 = Always   4 = Most of the time   3 = Half of the time   4 = Rarely   1 = Never

1. Did the student show concern for the patient's comfort and ensure privacy during the examination? 5 4 3 2 1
2. Did the student present himself/herself in a professional manner? 5 4 3 2 1
3. Did the student explain procedures and prepare the patient for what was being done? 5 4 3 2 1
4. Did the student perform the examination in a logical sequence, progressing from one region to another without repetition? 5 4 3 2 1
5. Did the student examine and compare symmetrical parts of the body? 5 4 3 2 1
6. Did the student use jargon not understood by the patient? 5 4 3 2 1
7. Was the examination too rough? 5 4 3 2 1

From: Katz FM and Snow R: Assessing Health Workers' Performance: A Manual for Training and Supervision. Geneva, Switzerland: World Health Organization, 1980, p. 135.

Table 7.4
Sample Questions for Feedback Following Discussion

DISCUSSION FEEDBACK SURVEY

1. To what extent did you feel part of the discussion group?
   A. Completely
   B. Often
   C. Sometimes
   D. Never

2. Was the group successful in getting out ideas and opinions on the topic?
   A. Highly
   B. Reasonably
   C. Partially
   D. Not at all

3. To what extent did the topic interest you?
   A. Very interested
   B. Somewhat interested
   C. Little interested
   D. Not interested

4. How did the group leader behave?
   A. Did most of the talking
   B. Did a lot of talking
   C. Did a moderate amount of talking
   D. Did little talking

   A. Encouraged others to do most of the talking
   B. Allowed a sizeable amount of group discussion
   C. Allowed some expression by others
   D. Did not allow others to express themselves

5. How would you rate the overall effectiveness of this discussion?
   A. Excellent
   B. Good
   C. Fair
   D. Poor

6. Comments

From: Whitman N: Discussion Feedback Questionnaire. Salt Lake City, UT: University of Utah Medical Center, Department of Family and Community Medicine. Reprinted by permission.

Instructors are wise to conduct a series of progress tests or formative evaluation events before they give students the final or summative test. In testing student competencies informally and frequently, instructors will know what dimensions of the teaching program pose difficulties, are poorly understood; or require further elucidation, practice, or review.

Since instructors require close to perfect student performance with respect to essential clinical prevention skills, it is doubly important to be sure that students are able to perform the subtle often complex procedures according to the criteria set by the instructor.

DELIVERING COURSES--SOME LESSONS LEARNED FROM THE KELLOGG PROJECT

Since 1975 the Center for Educational Development in Health at Boston University in collaboration with ATPM has been developing a competency-based instructional system on clinical prevention.[8] The project has been funded by the W.K. Kellogg Foundation since 1979. Project staff learned that the first few times an instructor gives a course some fine tuning of the content is required. Students may require more time for an exercise than originally planned; they may want the instructor to develop an example more completely; they may not understand the analytic methods described in an article and require an explanation.

The CEDH/ATPM instructional system Health Maintenance in Clinical Practice[8] was based on a performance analysis of practicing physicians and nurses previously mentioned.[4] Physicians and nurses who responded to the performance analysis through a Delphi Survey[9] indicated that their competencies were insufficient with respect to:

- analyzing the applicability of epidemiologic research results having to do with prevention and risk reduction;
- planning and managing preventive services;
- implementing behavioral components of health maintenance/ risk reduction programs with patients/clients.

The three project modules "The Epidemiologic Basis of Clinical Prevention," "Management for Preventive Services," and "Clinical Health Maintenance" were developed to address these needs. A performance analysis, even a quick and dirty one, yields invaluable dividends in structuring courses and curriculum in prevention.

In line with the experience that active learning yields optimal results, the project has developed cases and exercises for the three modules to encourage problem solving on the part of the student. Instructor's Manuals have also been developed. These provide options to the teacher in planning courses, seminars, and workshops.

In field testing early versions of the materials instructors requested that the authors provide the conceptual framework and protocols for each of the modules. As a result, extensive changes were made. In the published version the knowledge basis is supplied by means of textual materials, references, and outstanding articles/reports. Practical how-to-do-it guidelines are included for each clinical initiative. (See Chapter 8. Health Maintenance in Clinical Practice: An Annotated Review and Table 8.1.)

DISSEMINATING AN INNOVATIVE INSTRUCTIONAL SYSTEM

Because development of instructional materials is only half of the battle, the project has taken pains to choose eight model teaching centers in the U.S. where those interested in developing clinical prevention courses may turn for practical advice and encouragement. Each of our model teaching sites includes both schools of medicine and nursing which are cooperating in teaching their students clinical prevention. Model teaching sites include:

> University of Utah
> Pennsylvania State University/Hershey Medical Center
> University of Rochester
> University of California at San Diego
> Loma Linda University
> University of Iowa
> University of Nebraska
> SUNY/Health Science Center at Syracuse

These model teaching sites have all agreed to use Kellogg Project materials to plan new preventive medicine courses and to revise ones presently being offered. The cooperating sites were chosen on the basis of:

- present strength in preventive medicine teaching;
- interest in applying project-related initiatives;
- willingness to incorporate vertical and horizontal integration into the curriculum (see Figures 7.1 and 7.2);
- strong indication of support from the Dean's office;
- geographic representation.

The Dissemination Phase of the Project began April 1, 1985 although preliminary work was initiated half a year earlier. Some of the model teaching centers are presently beginning to set up clinical sites for their teaching. Courses involving physicians and nurses are also being initiated. The level of enthusiasm is high. To maintain the momentum, frequent meetings and ongoing consultation are planned. Institutionalization of the teaching program, periodic revision, and updating is of course the objective.

The Kellogg Project's Dissemination Strategy calls for a mix of enthusiastic people, time, and good materials. Altogether they yield a critical mass of activity.[10] The strategy might be summarized as follows:

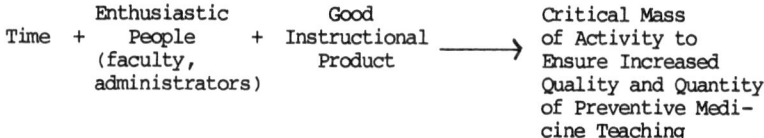

Time + Enthusiastic People (faculty, administrators) + Good Instructional Product → Critical Mass of Activity to Ensure Increased Quality and Quantity of Preventive Medicine Teaching

Enthusiastic people are needed to model good teaching in clinical prevention. Visitors to a health science center will be much more impressed by what they see being taught than by descriptive articles. Word will get around about successful teachers and their programs—and the programs will be emulated.

Time is needed. Instructors, especially in health professional schools, are slow in changing direction. Where curriculum committees, precedents, firmly ensconsed procedures hold sway it is difficult to make changes quickly.

A good product is essential. The American consumer is successful in resisting sales messages unless accompanied by a first rate product useful for his or her purposes. The product here includes instructional materials: cases, exercises, audio-visuals, tests created at the university or health science center, or adapted from published and unpublished sources. A superior product requires meticulous planning. The instructor(s) thinks through/discusses each activity. The instructor(s) allows sufficient time for each event as well as for questions and feedback from partici-pants.

These three components when put together will result in a snowball effect, in this case an increase in the quality and quantity of preventive medicine teaching.

SUMMARY

The teaching of clinical prevention focuses on a range of skills involving communicating effectively, clearly and dispassionately with the patient; interpreting complex and sophisticated laboratory tests; and applying behavior modification protocols. Trainees should also be able to analyze the cutting edge study such as the role of cholesterol in cardiovascular disease, use systems analysis skills to develop a flow chart for organizing a preventive service, develop computer files for each patient to allow review of preventive status and determination of what preventive protocols are required.

Such skills are only rarely taught today in the nation's health professions schools. We believe that such training is needed, that training methods and techniques are available and that, most important, the primary providers acknowledge their present deficiencies in this field and call for better teaching of prevention in the schools.

If the procedures for planning, implementing, and evaluating courses and practica in clinical prevention are applied, Cinderella will go to the ball in all her splendor. We will see yet another example of the unique ability of American health professions education to transform itself to meet the challenge of medicine and society.

REFERENCES

1. Kleinman JC: The Potential Impact of Risk Factor Modification on Coronary Heart Disease. Mortality in Middle-Aged Men. IN: Healthy People: The Surgeon General's Report on Health Promotion and Disease Prevention, Background Papers. Washington, DC: US Department of Health and Human Services, 1979, 187-195.

2. Ravenholt RT: Tobacco's impact on twentieth century U.S. mortality patterns. Amer J Prevent Med 1985;1(4):4-17.

3. Bok D: Needed: A new way to train doctors. Harvard Magazine, May-June 1984: 32-43, 70-71. ©1984 Harvard Magazine. Reprinted by permission.

4. Segall A, Barker W, et al.: A general model for preventive intervention in clinical practice. J Med Educ 1981;56:324-332.

5. Valente C, Sobal J, et al.: Health promotion, physician's beliefs, attitudes and practices. Amer J Prevent Med 1982;2(2):82-88.

6. Jonas S: Implementing the Recommendations of the GPEP Report Pertaining to Preventive Medicine. Washington, DC: Association of Teachers of Preventive Medicine, January 1986:1-25.

7. Segall A, Vanderschmidt H, Burglass R, Frostman T: Systematic Course Design in the Health Fields. New York: John Wiley, 1975.

8. Segall AJ and Vanderschmidt HF (eds.): Health Maintenance in Clinical Practice. Boston: Boston, University, Center for Educational Development in Health, 1985.

9. Linstone HA, Turoff M: The Delphi Method: Techniques and Applications. Reading, MA: Addison Wesley Publication Co., 1975.

10. Vanderschmidt H, Segall AJ: An instructional system as change agent. J Instructional Develop 1985;8(1):18-21.

CHAPTER 8
Health Maintenance in Clinical Practice: An Annotated Review
Victoria Logan Lamberton, B.A.

Health Maintenance in Clinical Practice[1] is an innovative, competency-based instructional series for students, teachers, and practicing health professionals. It comprises three modules: The Epidemiologic Basis of Clinical Prevention, Management for Preventive Services, and Clinical Health Maintenance. This series is a product of the Project for Curriculum Development in Preventive Medicine, supported by the W.K. Kellogg Foundation. The Center for Educational Development in Health (CEDH) of Boston University, in cooperation with The Association of Teachers of Preventive Medicine (ATPM), have conducted the project since 1977.

For each topic in the Instructional System (Table 8.1), there is a guidebook and an instructor's manual. The guidebooks are designed to provide the most important substantive information required for an understanding of the topic. The units include definitions, readings, questions, learning activities, exercises, case histories, and references. The guidebooks may serve as handbooks for primary care practices implementing preventive initiatives as well as guides for students.

The instructor's manuals provide a variety of suggestions for presenting the material on each topic, objectives, answers to selected questions posed in cases and exercises, suggestions for evaluation, and administrative data (eg, approximate time requirements for classroom teaching, preparation and/or practice).

This review contains annotations for the guidebook units only.

MODULE I: THE EPIDEMIOLOGIC BASIS OF CLINICAL PREVENTION: GUIDEBOOK

Module I sets forth principles of descriptive and analytic epidemiology, epidemiologic surveillance and intervention trials, as they apply to providing preventive care in clinical practice. Specific applications include critical appraisal of effectiveness of preventive interventions; planning preventive services for a defined practice population; assessing health and risk status; and monitoring effectiveness of preventive care.

Table 8.1
**CEDH/ATPM Curriculum Development Project Instructional Series:
Health Maintenance in Clinical Practice**

THE INSTRUCTIONAL SYSTEM: AN OVERVIEW

The Instructional System consists of 3 <u>Modules</u>:

I. The Epidemiologic Basis of Clinical Prevention

II. Management for Preventive Services

III. Clinical Health Maintenance

    Volume 1. Concepts and Methods
    Volume 2. Smoking
    Volume 3. Hypertension
    Volume 4. Nutritional Aspects of Cardiovascular Disease
    Volume 5. Immunization
    Volume 6. Cancer of the Breast
    Volume 7. Occupational Health

EACH MODULE COMPRISES

──────────── TWO COMPONENTS ────────────

GUIDEBOOK:	<u>Methods and procedures</u> for use in case studies, patient simulations and clinical encounters	INSTRUCTOR'S MANUAL:	Recommended learning activities, answers to selected questions, administrative data
	<u>Learning resources</u> - exercises, case studies		
	<u>Readings</u> - key papers and supplementary references		

This module contains four major sections (A - D), each subdivided into several units which develop specific aspects of the epidemiologic basis. Each unit includes a brief introduction with stated learning objectives and a series of learning activities (eg, lecture outlines, readings, films, and case studies).

Section A. Health (Three Units)

Section A raises provocative and philosophical challenges to the disease-oriented "health professions" to define, measure, and consider. Determinants and fundamental attributes of human well-being are discussed. One of the first readings contains a glossary of terms. The approach to Section A is attitudinal and motivational.

UNIT 1. THE DEFINITION OF HEALTH: ITS DIMENSIONS AND DETERMINANTS

Unit 1 explores the concept of health and its many aspects, surveying historical and contemporary views. It includes potential health attainments late in life, and explanations for prolongation of life expectancy. It introduces views of health which emanate from film, literature, and social science writing, including case histories. The goal is to enable the reader to identify appropriate dimensions and determinants of health and to develop a personal definition of health, more than just "the absence of disease".

UNIT 2. HEALTH STATUS

Unit 2 reviews basic concepts about health status within various frames of reference, eg, anatomic, functional, adaptive, and subjective. The unit develops an approach to health assessment through observation and self-report. Activities involve interviewing people both in and outside of health care settings to formulate assessment criteria. Guidelines for collecting the data are given. The goal is to enable the reader/interviewer to give a rough assessment of the health of the respondent based on the dimensions and determinants of health as reported verbally and/or observed.

UNIT 3. HEALTH PROMOTION

Unit 3 outlines criteria for the development of health promotion strategies at the level of practice. The focus is on the individual rather than the population. Factors influencing successful outcome of behavior change, health promotion efforts, and aspects of the provider-patient relationship are discussed. Given a case history, the goal is to assess the advisability and likely effectiveness of health promotion intervention.

Section B. Risk and the Natural History of Disease (Three Units)

Section B introduces basic concepts needed for an understanding of prevention of disease. It provides a practical model for illustrating the place of risk factors in one's conceptual thinking about the occurrence of disease and opportunities for intervention. Measurement and reduction of risk in the individual are discussed, primarily using examples from the fields of cardiovascular disease and cancer. Some methodological issues interspersed in this section are helpful preparation for Section C.

UNIT 4. THE NATURAL HISTORY OF DISEASE

Unit 4 presents the paradigm of the natural history of disease and refines this concept with the concept of staging. Visual portrayal of the model, showing potential health service interventions, is included. Graphics and activities focus on atherosclerosis/coronary heart disease (CHD) and cancer as examples. Suggested activities include films, panel discussion, and field study-patient interviews, visits to health care facilities, and graphic presentation of descriptive statistics. Given suitable reading material on a disease, the goal is to describe it in natural-history-of-disease format, projecting the impact on a patient at different points; to interpret simple epidemiologic tables and graphs; and to explain the terms incidence, prevalence, and person years of observation.

UNIT 5. MEASURING RISK

Unit 5 describes risk and characteristics of risk which make anecdotal evidence alone insufficient to confirm an association: low incidence of most diseases, small risk estimates, long latency period, multiple causes. The unit discusses measurement of risk in populations (relative risk, attributable risk) and in individuals. It presents two case histories with the goal that the reader will assess CHD risk and explain how risk factors might be derived. Attention is given to environmental and social factors.

UNIT 6. RISK REDUCTION

Unit 6 defines health and risk status modification, and outlines rules for disease prevention through risk reduction, including examples under primary and secondary prevention. The unit lists questions to consider in analyzing reports of risk reduction programs in the literature, and assessing their effectiveness. Three case histories are presented covering moderate-high risk for CHD; primary, secondary, and tertiary prevention. Here the goal is for readers to describe appropriate preventive interventions, considering the patient's stage of disease, and to estimate probable efficacy of intervention.

Section C. Assessment of Epidemiologic Evidence (Seven Units)

Section C begins with a brief review of basic terminology and methodology of descriptive and analytic epidemiology and intervention trials. Suggested readings from the medical literature largely draw upon studies with a relevance to clinical practice rather than public health. Extensive cross-references to major introductory epidemiology texts are included. (This section may, in many instances, serve as a brief refresher for persons who have already completed a formal epidemiology course.)

HEALTH MAINTENANCE IN CLINICAL PRACTICE: AN ANNOTATED REVIEW

The purpose of Section C is to teach the assessment of evidence related to prevention. It encourages readers to find answers to two fundamental questions: What kind of relationship exists between a particular risk factor and a given disease? What evidence do we have that specific behaviors or interventions are really preventive measures? The tools used are those of epidemiology with some assistance from biostatistics.

The seven sessions are organized to meet two objectives on the part of the reader: to be able to read and understand epidemiological studies of various kinds and to become familiar with some of the issues involved in relating the findings from epidemiological studies to the practice of clinical prevention.

UNIT 7. READING THE LITERATURE

Unit 7 outlines types of studies on human subjects: descriptions (clinical, epidemiological); analyses of nature (observational)—classified along the time dimension or according to the sampling frame; and experimental manipulation (four levels of specificity). The unit presents guidelines (seven rules) for critique of a medical report and diagrams ways of studying a disease: prospective, retrospective, and cross-sectional. The goal is to be able to evaluate an article from the literature in a systematic manner.

UNIT 8. DESCRIPTIVE STUDIES

Unit 8 discusses two kinds of descriptive study: the clinical description and the epidemiological description. It presents rules for each: for the description of the natural history of a disease, and for a descriptive epidemiologic study (focussing on age, sex, race, and social status variables). Activities feature articles on rheumatic fever/rheumatic heart disease and geographic patterns of breast cancer in the U.S. Given articles from the literature, the goal is to identify and interpret descriptive studies, explain how they differ from other studies, define epidemiologic terms used, and describe the comparisons presented.

UNIT 9. ANALYTIC STUDIES: CROSS-SECTIONAL

Unit 9 reviews the classification of studies along dimensions of time and sampling frame. Cross-sectional study (or prevalence survey) is described and contrasted to incidence study. The activity focuses on an article on hypertension screening. The goal is to interpret and describe the advantages of cross-sectional studies.

UNIT 10. ANALYTIC STUDIES: CASE CONTROL

Unit 10 presents concepts and rules pertaining to case control studies, including reference to advantages, disadvantages, relative risk, the art of selecting controls, measurement bias, and confounding. Given reports of case control studies, the goal is for the reader to explain how they differ from other analytic epidemiological studies, discuss advantages and disadvantages of this type of design, and interpret study results.

178 HANDBOOK OF CLINICAL PREVENTION

UNIT 11. ANALYTIC STUDIES: COHORTS, EXPOSED/UNEXPOSED

Unit 11 discusses procedures, problems, and advantages associated with studies of exposed versus unexposed and studies of cohorts. The activity uses Doll's[2] study of mortality from lung cancer in asbestos workers. Reference is made to the Doll and Hill[3] study of mortality and smoking among British physicians and to the Framingham Study.[4] Given representative cohort studies, the goal is for the reader to describe advantages and disadvantages of the cohort approach, use the concept of person years, and interpret and evaluate sample studies.

UNIT 12. EXPERIMENTAL STUDIES: CLINICAL TRIALS AND FIELD TRIALS

Unit 12 presents concepts of effectiveness, efficacy, and efficiency, with reference to clinical and field experiments. The MRFIT program (Multiple Risk Factor Intervention Trial)[5] and Rose et al's[6] randomized controlled trial of anti-smoking advice are the basis of learning activity. The unit outlines criteria for unbiased comparison in clinical trials and issues to be raised in discussing life style interventions. On finishing this unit, the reader should be able to describe the elements in representative experimental studies, interpret, and evaluate them.

UNIT 13. QUALITY OF EVIDENCE

Unit 13 presents the concept of necessary and sufficient conditions to dismiss discussion of whether an agent is _the_ cause of a disease, to illustrate the relation to host and environment, and to explain the strength of epidemiology as compared to clinical medicine in its ability to seek for sufficient cause (by means of community study). The unit outlines criteria for assessing the likelihood that a given association is causal. The activity involves critique of papers on the relationship of smoking to coronary heart disease. The goal is for readers to be able to evaluate the quality of the evidence presented in representative articles from the literature.

Section D. Meeting Population Needs (Three Units)

This section concludes the module with a series of activities that involve analyzing data from various primary care practice settings and populations with the goal of planning and implementing clinical preventive services. It draws upon the content of the preceding sections to provide the tools for informed decision making in one's practice. This in turn anticipates the detailed development of "Management for Preventive Services" and "Clinical Health Maintenance" which are the themes of Modules II and III.

Health professionals who are about to enter into practice should find these units particularly useful. Any reader familiar with the vocabulary of medicine/preventive health care and who has a modest understanding of epidemiology and statistics (eg, having completed Section C of this module) will be able to appreciate this section.

HEALTH MAINTENANCE IN CLINICAL PRACTICE: AN ANNOTATED REVIEW 179

UNIT 14. MEETING POPULATION NEEDS: SELECTING A PRACTICE SITE

Unit 14 focuses on the use of available demographic and health data in the selection of a practice. Rules for describing practice populations are presented. The reading, activities, and guiding questions in this unit help the reader to develop a logical basis for selecting a place to practice, using actual demographic/socioeconomic, public health, and medical care data.

UNIT 15. MEETING POPULATION NEEDS: SCREENING FOR UNRECOGNIZED ILLNESS

Unit 15 explicates methods for detecting previously unrecognized illness in the population. It outlines criteria for the evaluation of a screening test (including validity--sensitivity and specificity; yield--predictive value) and rules for the conduct of screening programs (with mention of mass screening, case finding, the periodic health examination). Given a proposal to screen a specified practice population for one or more diseases, the goal is for the reader to be able to discuss the pros and cons.

UNIT 16. MEETING POPULATION NEEDS: EVALUATION OF THE PREVENTIVE PROGRAM

Unit 16 demonstrates a simple approach to evaluating the extent to which a preventive program meets the needs of the relevant population. Guidelines and exercises geared for those planning to start a practice are offered to enable them to define preventive goals for the practice in measurable terms and establish routine data collections to assess progress toward those goals in a given practice setting.

MODULE II: MANAGEMENT FOR PREVENTIVE SERVICES: GUIDEBOOK (Seven Units)

Module II presents concepts of management and guidelines for implementing preventive initiatives in primary care practice. Health care providers as well as students should find the procedures outlined in this module useful in planning or modifying preventive services. The learning resources include cases from the Harvard Business School's Intercollegiate Case Clearing House and a set of practice descriptions.

The Module II Guidebook is organized according to a logical process which can be followed by providers who want to implement a preventive initiative (Figure 8.1). Unit 1 discusses the organization forms to be found in medical practices. The application of any of the management schemes which follow are to be tailored to the organizational form of a specific primary care practice. Unit 2 covers the preventive initiatives which primary care practices might offer.

For initiatives which significantly influence practice management, analysis of the implementing process is recommended. Analysis proceeds through the development of a protocol, the assignment of staff and community resources, and an estimate of how income will develop to allow the

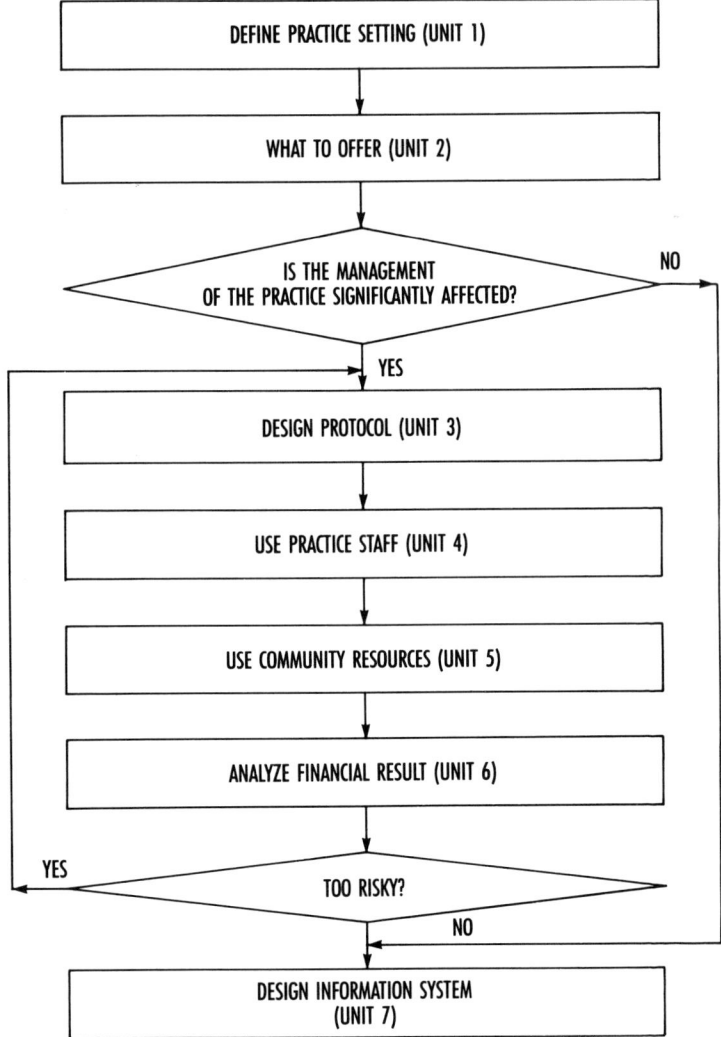

Figure 8.1. How the Module II Guidebook can be used to implement a preventive initiative. Skip Units 3 through 6 if the initiative does not have significant impact on the management of the practice. Recycle if financial analysis suggests an unacceptable risk for the practice.

practice to support the preventive initiative. If, on the basis of the analysis, it appears that the implementation of the initiative is too risky, the analyst must go "back to the drawing board," modifying the protocol and staffing pattern until a sufficiently risk free approach emerges.

UNIT 1. ORGANIZATION AND OBJECTIVES OF MEDICAL PRACTICE

Unit 1 introduces practice management, including setting objectives, in relation to the type of practice. Solo, group, and institutional forms and collaborative (eg, nurse practitioner/physician) aspects of practice are discussed, considering the interactions among staff and patients associated with each. A series of practice descriptions and detailed questionnaires which define each practice type are included. Activities in this unit should enable readers to identify the elements which characterize each form of practice and to explain the ways in which practices differ from models of the organization forms. Finally, the reader is asked to set objectives given this understanding of practice types. "Management by Objective" (MBO) techniques are described in the reading selection.

UNIT 2. WHAT TO OFFER

Unit 2 discusses the preventive initiatives which primary care practices might offer. Such initiatives are categorized by primary/secondary prevention, by frequency of patient assessment, and according to whether they require a significant modification of the management of the practice (ie, require new personnel, additional facilities, substantial staff training or staff time to implement and maintain the initiative).

This unit presents examples of preventive initiatives likely to require significant modification of the practice management, listing for each initiative the population at risk, assessment method, and intervention. Initiatives in secondary prevention, including many which would not require significant changes in management approach, or changes only in the practice's information systems, are covered in a reading selection.

Finally, using examples and exercises, the unit develops criteria which allow a practitioner to decide which initiatives a given practice might undertake. These criteria include objective considerations such as practice specialty and patient population along with subjective considerations such as the skills and interests of the practice staff.

UNIT 3. HOW TO DESIGN PATIENT FLOW PATTERNS (PROTOCOLS)

Unit 3 discusses advantages of using explicit protocols to manage patient care: allowing the identification and organization of personnel and community resources to help the practitioner meet patient needs, and allowing the organization of an effective information system. This unit outlines the flow charting process. The outcome is a diagram indicating the actions and decisions to be made in dealing with a patient who is a candidate for a protocol. The flow charted protocol is presented as a means of organizing resources and aiding communication.

The activity in this unit involves choosing a preventive initiative—smoking, hypertension, or diet—and developing a protocol in the form of a flow chart for one of the practice descriptions in Unit 1. Step-by-step instructions are included. The example traces a flow chart for a smoking cessation program in a solo or small group practice.

UNIT 4. HOW TO STAFF

Unit 4 addresses the problem of staffing to handle the protocols developed in Unit 3, where the practice plans to provide services through its own operation. Readings and activities lead the reader to consider staffing decisions which will maximize the appropriate use of physicians, nurses, physician assistants, clinical psychologists, health educators, nutritionists, and secretary/receptionists, in implementing preventive initiatives. Cost effectiveness, time, and the ability to understand and motivate patients are taken into account.

This unit suggests a methodical approach to the selection of personnel by identifying personnel resources available within the practice and those which can be hired from the community; these personnel are then matched to the various activities and decisions defined by the protocols developed in Unit 3. Factors which affect hiring decisions include the size of the practice and whether it is in a rural or an urban setting.

The reader is asked to make recommendations for staffing the protocols developed earlier in flow chart form. An example, including personnel resource chart and organizational chart for a small private practice, is provided.

UNIT 5. COMMUNITY RESOURCES

This unit discusses in general terms the use of community resources by a practice which wishes to refer a patient for a service that is part of a preventive initiative. Key aspects of referral—a good understanding of the service, some feedback on the patient's progress, and evaluation of the service—are addressed. Some suggestions are provided on the kind of services which may exist in the community and ways of finding them.

Activities in this unit refer back to protocols developed in Unit 3 for particular preventive initiatives. Readers are asked to identify and evaluate available community resources that might be used for a variety of interventions (eg, weight loss, smoking cessation, stress control, and alcohol/drug abuse prevention programs).

The example features referral for smoking cessation by a pediatric nurse practitioner who manages the maternal and child health clinic at a city hospital. A checklist of questions and criteria to evaluate smoking cessation programs is included.

UNIT 6. HOW TO PLAN FOR INCOME FROM PREVENTIVE SERVICES

This unit develops some analytical tools which allow the reader to determine the impact of adding a preventive initiative to the services offered by the practice when the initiative will have a significant impact on the management of the practice. The approach identifies the cost of the initiative to the practice, estimates the income the practice will receive from the initiative, and determines what financial risk is involved in offering the preventive initiative. The resulting analysis allows the practice to make a rational decision on offering the preventive initiative or, should the risk be too high, modifying the protocol to reduce the risk to an acceptable level.

Third-party coverage of services provided in an outpatient, fee-for-service setting and in certain other settings is discussed. Activities in this unit incorporate protocols, staff assignments, and community resource information from previous units. Readers are asked to calculate the cost, income, and risk of introducing a preventive initiative, given step-by-step guidelines. The example gives an analysis based on the practice first described in Unit 4.

UNIT 7. INFORMATION SYSTEMS

The use of information systems to support preventive initiatives is discussed. The design of information systems is approached from a computer science viewpoint, although granting that a practice may choose to implement a manual system initially. Data collection is based on the protocol developed in Unit 3 and the staffing decisions made in Units 4 and 5. Computer science methods are used to enter the data to be recorded and to produce reports. The techniques presented are useful for both preventive interventions which do and those which do not have significant impact on practice management.

The activity and the example in this unit give guidelines for developing an information system to fit a specific preventive protocol. The readings describe an information system designed for a hospital and a program developed for use in preventive medical care.

MODULE III: CLINICAL HEALTH MAINTENANCE—GUIDEBOOKS

Module III focuses on acquisition of technical and interpersonal skills in preventive assessment and intervention, as they apply to the control of selected health hazards, diseases, and conditions. It outlines screening protocols and preventive procedures appropriate for the practice of health maintenance in clinical settings.

The module is divided into seven volumes. Volume 1, Concepts and Methods, presents a general algorithm for clinical health maintenance, as shown in Figure 8.2. The numbers in parentheses correspond to the units (1-10) in this guidebook. The algorithm sets a pattern for sub-

184 HANDBOOK OF CLINICAL PREVENTION

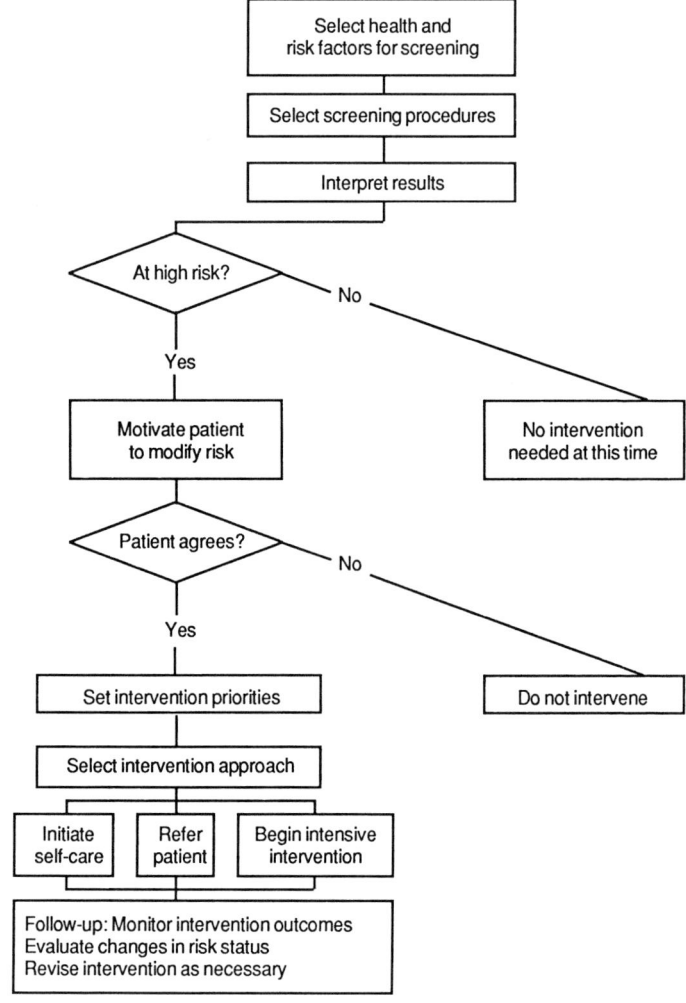

Figure 8.2. General clinical health maintenance algorithm.

sequent volumes, in which preventive initiatives for specific health hazards and conditions are discussed.

Volume 1: Concepts and Methods (Ten Units)

UNIT 1. INITIAL SCREENING FOR HEALTH AND RISK STATUS

Unit 1 defines health and risk and presents concepts and procedures for assessing health and risk status for different age groups. Assessment is discussed in the context of normal clinical practice, as a basis for disease prevention/health promotion interventions. The unit describes a Health and Risk Oriented Patient History, summarizing the main points to be addressed in matrix form. An example of a self-administered questionnaire is included.

UNIT 2. SELECTING SCREENING PACKAGES AND PROCEDURES

Unit 2 gives guidelines for age- and sex-specific screening. Included are criteria and general procedures for screening/case finding of conditions, diseases, and risk factors which can be prevented or detected at an early stage. The screening packages, presented in tabular form, were adapted from recommendations by Frame and Carlson,[7] Breslow and Somers,[8] the Canadian Task Force,[9] and the American Cancer Society.[10] Guidelines for pregnant women, infants, children, adults, and older adults are listed. Activities, readings, and additional resources discuss coronary heart disease (CHD) and cancer risks, among others.

UNIT 3. INTERPRETING RESULTS OF HEALTH AND RISK APPRAISAL

Unit 3 describes health hazard/health risk appraisal systems (HHAs, HRAs) and gives several examples of assessment instruments, computerized and noncomputerized, showing how they can be interpreted. HHAs by Farquhar,[11] the American Heart Association,[12] and the Centers for Disease Control[13] are included. The strengths and weaknesses of these risk factor/health hazard appraisal systems are discussed. Readers are asked to evaluate the instruments by answering a series of questions. A sample print-out for "I'm a Health Nut,"[14] an HRA designed for adolescents to increase their awareness of health needs and behaviors, also appears in this unit.

UNIT 4. MOTIVATING THE PATIENT

This unit discusses theories and methods used to motivate people for behavior change and risk reduction. The focus is on preparing reluctant or unmotivated patients to participate in behavior change programs. Maslow's[15] and McClelland's[16] concepts of motivation are presented.

The goal is for the reader to be able to discuss motivation as an element of behavior change; to describe some recognized approaches to the problem; and to apply accepted techniques in motivating people to participate/comply, particularly in CHD prevention programs. Guidelines, examples, and a role play situation are provided.

186 HANDBOOK OF CLINICAL PREVENTION

UNIT 5. SETTING INTERVENTION PRIORITIES

This unit outlines the components of a successful patient-provider negotiation to select one or more conditions for intervention, based on the results of risk assessment and health appraisal. The discussion emphasizes the importance of timely intervention and choosing risk factors that can be changed, ie, for which behavior change is feasible and practical.

Five general steps in setting intervention priorities are presented. By the end of the negotiation process, the patient and provider will have discussed the risk factors, selected one or two for further consideration, estimated patient interest, reviewed past efforts at behavior change, and set behavioral goals within his/her current abilities.

This unit also suggests a project to modify another individual's CHD risk. Beginning with procedures described in Units 1 through 4, the project continues through the last unit of the guidebook, "Monitoring and Evaluating the Outcomes of Intervention."

UNIT 6. SELECTING AN INTERVENTION APPROACH

Unit 6 discusses four basic approaches to behavior change, describing the major features of each (self-care, self-directed, group-supported, professionally-directed/individualized). A three-step procedure is outlined for selecting the strategy most appropriate to patient style and the risk factor to be modified. Emphasis is placed on the importance of allocating time to discuss alternative approaches and to clarify the roles of the provider and patient in the intervention process.

The tables in this unit present patient and provider variables favoring selection of a particular intervention approach and behavioral modalities used in the prevention of CHD and other conditions. Each approach is considered in terms of cost, time required, convenience, group or individual orientation, and effectiveness with various risk factors.

UNIT 7. THE PRIMARY CARE PROVIDER AND SELF-DIRECTED BEHAVIOR CHANGE

Unit 7 describes the basic principles associated with self-directed behavior change. Elements cited as critical to the success of this approach include assessment of readiness, hints to be given to a patient selecting this approach, and negotiation of the precise role of the primary health care provider in the process.

Warning patients of potential side effects is recommended to counteract the major limitation of the self-directed approach. Also recommended are dividing the goal into small, manageable segments and providing intermittent reinforcement. Using smoking cessation as an example, this unit lists published guides available from national organizations at little or no cost to help individuals implement behavior change.

HEALTH MAINTENANCE IN CLINICAL PRACTICE: AN ANNOTATED REVIEW   187

UNIT 8. THE PRIMARY CARE PROVIDER AND REFERRAL FOR BEHAVIOR CHANGE

Unit 8 describes concepts of referral to community groups for behavior change. Included are detailed criteria (eg, patient preference, financial resources, program availability) and recommended steps for referral. The goal is to enable providers, through an understanding of some of the dimensions of the group approach, to make the best match between patients and a behavior change group.

Making clear to the client the provider's responsibility and scheduling followup sessions are among the recommendations. To help implement referral, this unit provides a sample followup plan, questions to guide the evaluation of referral centers, and a table of group oriented techniques, by risk factor.

UNIT 9. THE PRIMARY CARE PROVIDER AND DIRECT INTERVENTION

Unit 9 describes implementation methods for direct (one-to-one) intervention for behavior change. The health maintenance contract is featured as the core of a behavior change program implemented within an ongoing primary health care provider-patient relationship. This unit overviews criteria for selecting the direct, individualized approach, steps in the development of a contract, as well as potential problems associated with this form of intervention.

The steps include exploring baseline data, developing a health maintenance plan, warning about potential side effects associated with the behavior change, and planning followup. A sample behavior change contract, guidelines for using other health team members in preventive efforts, and a table of individually oriented techniques (for selected risk factors) are provided.

UNIT 10. THE PROVIDER AND FOLLOWUP: MONITORING AND EVALUATING THE
         OUTCOMES OF INTERVENTION

Unit 10 summarizes the essential aspects of followup to ensure maintenance of behavior change. It describes strategies for tailoring followup to patient needs, outlines types of followup, and offers guidelines for modifying the original intervention plan.

The importance of continuous monitoring to evaluate compliance, check progress, and sustain reinforcement and motivation throughout the gradual process of health risk behavior change is emphasized. Suggestions for followup scheduling are included. The reader is asked to review experiences with each component of the intervention process and to make recommendations for patients in similar settings.

Volume 2: Smoking (Eight Units)

UNIT 1. INITIAL SCREENING AND INTERPRETING RESULTS

Unit 1 presents guidelines for screening for smoking as a risk factor (especially for coronary heart disease) and interpreting the results. All patients are considered candidates for screening; the recommended health message focuses on each patient's particular areas of concern. The assessment/counseling process as outlined in this unit covers smoking habits, related behavior, physical health, and specific cardiovascular information. The goal is to conduct a sensitive assessment, which will enable the provider and patient to decide on the most effective way to reduce the individual's health risk.

Suggested activities include discussion of the case histories contained in this volume and screening and counseling a volunteer "client" regarding smoking risk. A sample smoking questionnaire, daily smoking record, smoking graph, and smoker's self tests for adults and for young people are provided.

UNIT 2. HEALTH PROMOTION

Unit 2 directs the health promotion message to all patients but especially to young nonsmokers and high risk individuals. Suggested ways in which providers can influence patients not to smoke include setting a personal example, changing presenting complaints into a health message, offering verbal encouragement, and providing information about health risks and benefits. A personalized explanation of the advantages of not smoking is recommended as particularly effective. For young people, emphasis on immediate effects and resisting social pressures to smoke is advised.

Activities in this unit include practice interviews involving "clients" with various histories and presenting complaints and role play (or actual) health promotion-oriented assessments/interviews with junior and senior high school students.

UNIT 3. SETTING PRIORITIES TO REDUCE SMOKING RISK

Unit 3 outlines an approach to setting priorities in order to minimize smoking risk. Setting priorities is described as a cooperative process between the patient and the health care provider. Steps are recommended, including questions and factors to consider in using assessment data to arrive at a realistic plan.

This unit suggests that by taking time to determine the patient's interest in change, as well as past and current smoking behavior, the provider will be better able to suggest realistic, manageable goals. To this end, the provider is encouraged to convey a firm belief in the importance of minimizing smoking and to communicate the expectation of success. Using a case history and practice "clients," the reader is asked to develop and justify short-term and long-term goals to reduce smoking risk. Optional use of videotape.

UNIT 4. SELECTING AN INTERVENTION MODALITY

This unit describes the process of negotiating to select an intervention modality, with emphasis on the commitment of time and care which this involves. Three approaches are considered in light of patient and provider characteristics: change through self-direction, group support (referral), and primary health care provider intervention. Among the factors governing the selection are individual personalities/preferences, past experience, available time and resources, stage in the cessation effort, and the provider-client relationship. Agreement on an appropriate intervention strategy is the desired outcome.

This unit includes a table of patient and provider variables favoring particular intervention approaches for cessation/control of smoking. The table also can help define the two players' respective roles in the change process. Suggested activities involve case studies and/or continuation of practice counseling sessions begun in earlier units.

UNIT 5. SELF-DIRECTED CHANGE

Unit 5 focuses on the self-directed approach, with emphasis on individual responsibility for smoking behavior change. The importance of self-efficacy as a predictor of success is highlighted.

This unit describes the steps involved in self-directed smoking intervention, which requires the patient to set personal goals and to implement a behavior change plan, with limited professional involvement. The information presented will guide the primary health care provider in determining patient readiness, pointing to materials which suggest a manageable sequence of goals, and negotiating a precise role in the intervention strategy. Guidelines are given to assist the provider in motivating and reinforcing individuals who choose this approach and monitoring their progress.

Included is a discussion of potential side effects of smoking cessation and a list of smoking cessation aides available at little or no charge.

UNIT 6. REFERRAL TO OUTSIDE RESOURCE

Unit 6 reviews the main features of group-supported behavior change, in order to guide the provider in referring a would-be ex-smoker to an appropriate cessation program. Factors to consider in making such a referral include patient preference, financial and personal resources, plus the availability of suitable programs. The primary provider's role is to evaluate the program and monitor progress at regular intervals. The suggested activity involves searching the local community for smoking cessation groups (partial list of sponsors is provided), visiting and reporting on the characteristics (strengths/weaknesses) of one of them.

UNIT 7. PRIMARY CARE PROVIDER INTERVENTION

Unit 7 describes the process of planning, implementing, and monitoring a cessation program within the context of an ongoing provider-patient relationship. Steps include development of a behavior change contract (sample provided), discussion of potential problems associated with withdrawal, and outlining a followup plan.

Time and cost factors are discussed, as well as requirements for effective intervention (ie, support, encouragement, and information about alternatives, offered by the provider throughout an individual's smoking change effort). As part of this unit's activity, the reader is asked to examine goals and subgoals, and then to write a contract for behavior change, using case history data.

UNIT 8. FOLLOWUP: MONITORING/EVALUATING/REVISING

Unit 8 presents followup activities as equal in importance to the steps of assessing behavior, setting priorities, and choosing an intervention modality. It gives recommendations for scheduling patient contacts (for the purpose of monitoring behavior change), evaluating progress, and revising the intervention plan.

Included are a variety of mechanisms for followup and suggestions for evaluating discrepancies in current versus desired practice. In the activity, the reader can apply principles of followup to a specific case that was introduced earlier.

Volume 3: Hypertension (Seven Units)

UNIT 1. COLLECTING AND INTERPRETING ASSESSMENT DATA

Unit 1 sets the context for this volume: Although mortality from cardiovascular disease has declined, the challenge remains to prevent, detect, treat, and control high blood pressure. This unit examines hypertension, as a primary coronary heart disease risk factor, and the collection and interpretation of assessment data for the primary and secondary prevention of high blood pressure.

Definitions and detailed procedures for assessing adults and children, including physical examination and laboratory criteria, are presented. Activities call for analysis and discussion of the decline in cardiovascular disease mortality, classification of blood pressure levels from patient profile data, and demonstration/teaching/explanation of blood pressure measurement.

UNIT 2. SETTING INTERVENTION GOALS

Unit 2 describes the rationale behind both the primary and the secondary prevention of high blood pressure and outlines the major options available for preventive and treatment interventions. It also discusses the development of an intervention plan, involving negotiation of a partnership agreement between the practitioner and the patient to determine goals and set priorities for action.

The hygienic measures of weight control, regulation of lipid, sodium and potassium intake, exercise, stress reduction, and other factors associated with preventing or lowering high blood pressure, and the pharmacological stepped care approach to the treatment of essential hypertension, are addressed in this unit. For persons with normal blood pressures, attention to risk factor reduction also is recommended in view of growing evidence that the initial rise in blood pressure may be preventable, especially if preventive measures are instituted early in life.

Activities include preparing primary prevention recommendations for certain population groups; discussing "the preventive approach versus the medical approach" to high blood pressure; and devising a therapeutic plan, using the Stepped Care Approach (case histories provided in this volume).

UNIT 3. SETTING PRIORITIES AND SELECTING THE INTERVENTION

Unit 3 describes the intervention plan negotiation process between the patient and the provider that leads to the establishment of short- and long-term goals. The design of a health maintenance plan takes into account factors and behaviors that can influence adherence and outcome. The modes of implementation discussed are: self-care, referral for behavior change, and provider directed.

Criteria for establishing an intervention program are listed. Activities involve a simulated patient interview and writing a Health Maintenance Plan. A sample plan is provided (including risk factors, current and goal status, and means for achieving goals and measuring the level of achievement).

UNIT 4. IMPLEMENTING: SELF-CARE

Unit 4 directs recommendation for self-care to those patients with initiative, the ability to learn about their condition, and the willingness to take major responsibility for implementing and monitoring the intervention. This unit focuses on patient education, describing how to teach a patient about the causes, consequences, treatment, and prevention of high blood pressure. A detailed education protocol is included. This knowledge should enable the individual to execute the intervention plan with only minimal direction from the primary health care provider. The provider furnishes the patient with the necessary tools and materials for implementation, evaluates the outcome, and suggests modifications.

Most adult patients, as stated here, can be taught to measure their own behaviors related to high blood pressure (eg, monitoring body weight, caloric intake, salt intake, physical activity, sleep patterns, and stress coping techniques); however, they should be guided in the purchase of reliable instruments to measure blood pressure. Activities ask the reader to organize and write up a sample educational assessment; to review, critique, and evaluate hypertension patient education materials; and to design/implement a teaching program addressing CHD risk factor(s).

UNIT 5. IMPLEMENTING: REFERRAL FOR BEHAVIOR CHANGE

Unit 5 describes the criteria and procedures for referral for behavior change in primary and secondary prevention of high blood pressure. Referral as discussed here is to another professional or to a group for treatment or behavior change. Among the factors to consider are financial constraints, patient preference or prior positive experience with this mode of intervention, and the availability of particular services. The provider's responsibilities include the correct match of the patient to the referral, monitoring progress, and making any needed adjustments. Community agency assessment, according to specified criteria, is the subject of the suggested activities.

UNIT 6. IMPLEMENTING: PRIMARY CARE PROVIDER

This unit discusses the general responsibilities of the primary health care provider in the management of primary hypertension and its associated risk factors—obesity; lipid, sodium, and potassium consumption; physical fitness; and stress. The responsibilities include monitoring the patient's progress, maintaining the patient's adherence to the treatment program, and modifying the program if it fails to meet the patient's needs and the provider's expectations. A list of factors related to the patient and the provider, that may determine the degree of direct intervention, is presented.

The procedure includes cooperative development of a health maintenance plan. Provider responsibilities related to prevention and control of hypertension are detailed within the categories of planning, implementation, and evaluation. Suggested activities involve directing the pharmacological and behavioral management of a patient with hypertension (under supervision, or simulated via role play and/or case study).

UNIT 7. FOLLOWUP: MONITORING/EVALUATING/REVISING

Unit 7 presents followup as part of the implementation of the intervention plan, whether by self-care, referral, or carried out by the primary health care provider. Discussed are the elements of followup: monitoring progress and evaluating the treatment outcome for each patient, and revising the plan as needed. Included are strategies to monitor appointment-keeping behavior, improve adherence, followup and evaluate the outcome, and alter the intervention plan in the event that the anticipated outcome is not reached.

Sample reminder, record, and medication chart forms are provided. To achieve successful long-term maintenance treatment, this unit emphasizes the importance of a personal rapport between the individual participant and members of the health care staff. The activities incorporate program strategies to increase patient adherence to a regimen and practice the followup process.

Volume 4: Nutritional Aspects of Cardiovascular Disease (Seven Units)

UNIT 1. NUTRITIONAL SCREENING/INTERPRETING RESULTS

Unit 1 outlines the procedures used in screening and interpreting the primary and secondary nutrition risk factors in coronary heart disease. The criteria for assessing individual risk are presented in detail. The two major elements of the nutritional approach are cited: the preventive element (nutrition education) and the screening/treatment element.

Some of the procedures as described vary depending upon the individual's age and whether or not a family history of premature heart disease is present. The screening activities are intended to aid in identifying high-risk individuals who can be channeled into appropriate interventions.

This introductory section reviews the relationship of dietary variables, primary and secondary risk factors, and outcome in heart disease—diet/nutrition behavior change being featured as a major component of heart disease prevention. A number of definitions, for both this and subsequent units, are provided here. Activities refer to case study material which also is included.

UNIT 2. SETTING INTERVENTION GOALS AND PRIORITIES

Unit 2 describes the individual(client)-centered protocol for professional use in establishing realistic and specific goals and priorities for nutrition intervention. The process of setting short- and long-term goals for nutrition intervention (where needed) follows detailed nutrition assessment and definition of risk status.

A dietary and food behavior analysis and discussions between the professional and the client are recommended to determine the treatment plan, short-term treatment priorities, and the expected outcome of intervention. This usually requires rank ordering a number of problems, taking into account related behaviors and/or individual circumstances (case study included). The problems are tackled progressively during the intervention process.

This unit provides U.S. Dietary Goals/Guidelines; overall nutrition goals and dietary prescriptions in the prevention and treatment of heart disease, including an explanation of the American Heart Association three-phased approach; and a sample three-day dietary record.

UNIT 3. SELECTING AN INTERVENTION MODALITY

Unit 3 offers guidelines to assist the provider in choosing the best means of nutrition intervention to ultimately reduce or eliminate one or more of the risk factors associated with cardiovascular disease. Prior to selecting the strategy, the professional is advised to determine that the individual is, indeed, a motivated candidate, and to define the intervention priorities. Decision making then focuses on whether group, individual, or self-instructional treatment approaches are suitable.

The optimal outcome of choosing the proper nutrition intervention is described as permanent change in eating patterns, manifested over the long term by maintenance of ideal body weight, serum lipid levels, and blood pressure, and glucose tolerance. Emphasis is placed on the importance of personal commitment/assumption of responsibility by the client for health outcomes, gradual dietary modification in order to permanently change long-established habits, and agreement by the professional and the individual on intervention strategies. When the resources exist, it is recommended that the individual with a complicated nutrition disorder be referred to a registered dietician.

A suggested activity in this unit involves discussion of the complexity of variables that affect nutrition behavior. The following issues are addressed: length and goals of a counseling session, duration of counseling for behavior change, and family and community support systems for reinforcing appropriate client behavior. In addition, the reader is asked to compile a profile of the considerations in selecting different nutrition strategies.

UNIT 4. REFERRAL TO OUTSIDE RESOURCE

This unit describes resources which offer alternative modes of nutrition counseling. It also discusses the credibility of these resources, the criteria used in making referrals for nutrition care (eg, patient preference, provider time and training), and the nature (advantage and disadvantage) of these services.

Motivated individuals with complex nutrition or lipid disorders, or in need of long-term care, are recommended for referral to an outside nutrition professional or group. The responsibilities of the provider as outlined include assisting in the selection of credible nutrition resources that promote a balanced diet and follow procedures designed to make permanent changes in nutrition behavior, communicating treatment goals to outside professionals, monitoring individuals' progress, and recommending changes in protocol as needed.

The reader is invited to survey sources of nutrition counseling or therapy in the community. Questions and guidelines for critiquing these resources are provided.

UNIT 5. IMPLEMENTING THROUGH SELF-INSTRUCTION

Unit 5 focuses on self-guided nutrition care, which may be suitable for the person with an uncomplicated case and the ability to manage his/her dietary practices. The procedures outlined are useful in providing advice and guidance to individuals willing to assume personal responsibility for learning the principles of dietary behavior change and for developing an approach to their dietary intervention with minimal provider involvement.

The provider's responsibilities in this context can include identifying candidates for self-instruction, discussing the rationale and general principles of the diet, explaining the realistic outcomes of dietary change, assisting in setting personal health and nutrition goals, providing or referring the person to sources of nutrition information (eg, materials and other professionals), and monitoring and supporting progress on followup visits. Criteria for evaluating written nutrition resources are presented. The ideal outcome of nutrition intervention is described as permanent modification of eating habits, or a reinforcement of the person's present sound dietary regime, and long-term modification of nutritional risk factors.

UNIT 6. PROVIDER-BASED NUTRITION INTERVENTION

Unit 6 describes the provider's responsibility when assuming the role of the individual's primary nutrition counselor. The factors cited as key to success in this approach are a provider's expertise in nutrition, food, and counseling techniques, the client's motivation, and the provider's effectiveness in guiding the behavior change process. Having access to a nutrition professional, such as a registered dietician, for advice is recommended as the ideal situation. Suggested activities incorporate case studies, role play, and observation/practice interviewing and counseling.

The approach described in this unit is geared for those with the time, skill, and interest to offer in-depth nutrition counseling. General principles of nutrition interviewing are presented. With the individual's diet history as a guide, the provider begins by explaining the principles and rationale of dietary modification. Together, the professional and the client set goals and priorities for behavior change (examples listed) and agree on a time frame. The provider may furnish printed material that explains the diet and/or a list of references for further information. The individual is encouraged to keep a food diary for the purpose of evaluating compliance during followup visits. If the client does not shop for or prepare his/her own food, the person who shops and/or cooks is included in the counseling session.

UNIT 7. MONITORING AND EVALUATING OUTCOMES

This unit reviews the procedures of monitoring and evaluating the success of a nutrition intervention, as an integral component of the intervention/counseling process, regardless of the treatment modality selected. Monitoring addresses the individual's changes in dietary habits, level of interest/motivation, difficulties with behavior changes, and progress towards short- and long-term goals.

Discussed is the scheduling of followup visits for the individual involved in the behavior change process and mechanisms for monitoring progress (eg, dietary records; discussions with the professional; and measurements such as weight, blood pressure and serum lipid levels). Use of food records is recommended to indicate if the individual is achieving set goals and to help identify areas of adherence problems.

Follow-up sessions can sustain or provide motivation and lead to reestablishment of intervention goals, if needed. Active involvement of the individual, and if necessary, family members, in the monitoring and evaluation of diet intervention, is emphasized. If after sufficient time has elapsed, it is apparent that goals are not being reached, the provider is advised to consider a change in the mode of intervention. If the individual resists change, postponement or discontinuation of the intervention may be necessary.

Volume 5: Immunization (Five Units)

UNIT 1. COLLECTING AND INTERPRETING DATA

Unit 1 sets the context for this volume, addressing problems associated with public ignorance, inadequate medical record keeping, and inconsistent reporting guidelines, all of which can reduce the effectiveness of public and private immunization programs. The unit also presents definitions and procedures for organizing immunization data as a routine part of preventive health care.

Listed are commonly used vaccines and toxoids and preparations available for special use; as well as components of an immunization-related history. A form for reporting an adverse event following immunization and a list of additional sources of information are provided. Activities include immunization-related interviews and debate on the subject of legislation and health (eg, methods used by government agencies with respect to immunization).

UNIT 2. SELECTING AGENTS - ROUTINE COURSE

Unit 2 outlines schedules of immunization for normal infants and children and for individuals who have not been immunized routinely during infancy. A list of specific immunizing agents gives details of administration, indications, schedules, side effects, precautions, and contraindications associated with immunobiologics commonly in use. In addition, there are rules regarding the route and site of administration, technique, and dosage; and guidelines for shipment, handling, and storage of vaccines.

UNIT 3. SELECTING PATIENTS - ROUTINE COURSE

Unit 3 describes special factors to consider in planning immunization of particular groups of patients. It discusses deferment of immunizations in the presence of certain conditions, problems with regard to immunizing adults, vaccination during pregnancy, and hypersensitivity reactions to certain immunobiologics.

Four mini cases with questions are provided. Suggested activities also address the issue of preventing deficient immunizations at the workplace. Sources of further information are listed, including official package circulars supplied by the manufacturers of vaccines.

HEALTH MAINTENANCE IN CLINICAL PRACTICE: AN ANNOTATED REVIEW

UNIT 4. MOTIVATING AND EDUCATING PATIENTS AND PARENTS

This unit makes the case for better health education of adults, parents, and children, in order to help motivate the general public to take part in voluntary immunization programs. It also emphasizes the need to explain risks and benefits of vaccines and identifies barriers to proper immunization such as practitioner failure, vaccine failure, and social and behavioral variables. Examples of information, documents, and other means of motivating parents and patients to adhere to the immunization regimen are included, as well as one mini case with questions.

UNIT 5. INFORMATION SYSTEMS AND MANAGEMENT

Unit 5 gives guidelines for specific, personal followup, as well as accurate record keeping by providers and parents, which have been shown to increase the likelihood that the immunization course will be completed. Objectives of an immunization information (record keeping) system are outlined. Personal immunization cards distributed to parents of newborns and updated consistently are the key element of the information system. A corresponding office record is recommended to enable providers to keep track of the history and planned immunizations for each patient. Typical charts for pediatric and adult patients are provided.

Volume 6: Cancer of the Breast (Seven Units)

UNIT 1. COLLECTING AND INTERPRETING ASSESSMENT DATA

Unit 1 introduces the discussion of clinical breast cancer as consequent to several causes or factors acting in sequences. It reviews incidence and risk factor data for the United States, a family and/or personal history of breast cancer featured as less common and thus useful indicators of risk. Factors are listed according to high risk, low risk, and no firm relationship to risk. This unit outlines in detail the steps involved in taking a thorough history and performing breast examination, procedures described as critical in the evaluation of any signs or symptoms of breast disease.

UNIT 2. SETTING INTERVENTION GOALS

Unit 2 considers five broad types of interventions to prevent entirely or to diminish the mortality from breast cancer: nutrition counseling, reproductive counseling, preventive surgery, breast examination, and mammography. Three areas in which clinicians can counsel patients with expectation of diminishing the risk of breast cancer are discussed: nutrition, reproductive behavior, and preventive surgery. The three practical techniques presented for early detection of breast cancer, with absolute improved survival, are periodic breast examination by a health professional, breast self-examination by the patient, and mammography. Suggested activities include one mini case.

UNIT 3. SELECTING INTERVENTION MODALITIES

Unit 3 discusses practice and individual variables affecting the choice of intervention modalities. Nutrition counseling is described as potentially the most significant action clinicians can take which may eventually impact on breast cancer incidence and general health, therefore to be provided to all patients. Individual and community barriers to dietary change are listed, together with implications for practitioner action. A strategy for advocating dietary change in clinical practice also is provided.

Application of secondary preventive measures—breast examination and mammography—is recommended following careful consideration of several issues in individual patients as well as the priorities of the practice. The activities include one mini case with questions.

UNIT 4. IMPLEMENTING: SELF-CARE

Unit 4 outlines the specific content for educational programs directed to behaviors in four areas: nutrition, radiation limitation, breast self-examination, and decision making about mammography. Performing and teaching BSE (breast self-examination) is the subject of the activity in this unit. (Optional videotape)

UNIT 5. IMPLEMENTING: REFERRAL FOR BEHAVIOR CHANGE

Unit 5 gives guidelines for referral of patients as indicated for comprehensive nutrition counseling, genetic counseling, and instruction in breast self-examination. Referral for genetic counseling is advised in some cases when evaluation of a patient's history demonstrates a significant family history of cancer and, in particular, breast cancer. The discussion of genetic counseling of high risk individuals emphasizes the importance of establishing the specific history in the patient's family, through detailed medical records, including hospital discharge summaries, operative reports, pathology reports, and autopsy reports.

Assessment of patients' needs, desires, and expectations also is cited as important in preparing for a counseling session. A case example with calculation of risks is included.

UNIT 6. IMPLEMENTING: PHYSICIAN OR HEALTH PROVIDERS

Unit 6 considers briefly the importance of goals and strategies in the application of the preventive interventions proposed in earlier units. A table of goals, strategies, and potential obstacles to cancer prevention in clinical practice/early detection of breast cancer is presented. Algorithms for risk assessment, nutrition education, breast self-examination, mammography, and management of breast masses are detailed as a focus for discussion of the major questions clinicians must consider in implementing primary and secondary breast cancer preventive strategies.

HEALTH MAINTENANCE IN CLINICAL PRACTICE: AN ANNOTATED REVIEW

UNIT 7. FOLLOWUP: MONITORING, EVALUATING, REVISING

Unit 7 describes the team approach to the practice of clinical prevention of breast cancer, involving agreement on protocols and algorithms, and periodic evaluation of compliance with them. Extramural consultants are mentioned as playing a potentially useful role in auditing and educating the practice team. The suggested activity asks the reader to outline a system of followup for dietary counseling, with reference to a case presented in an earlier unit.

Volume 7: Occupational Health (Seven Units)

UNIT 1. OCCUPATIONAL HEALTH MONITORING AND SURVEILLANCE

Unit 1 sets the tone for the volume, which is written for the primary care health professional. The emphasis is on general skills that a health care provider needs when dealing with occupational health problems, including skills to find the necessary information.

This unit covers the strategies used to observe a population in order to detect occupational health problems (monitoring, surveillance, environmental monitoring). The basic principles described here apply to all situations in which screening is undertaken and to all diagnostic tests. Criteria for the selection of a screening test are presented. Extensive lists of non-profit services providing consultation on the evaluation of occupational exposures and illnesses (national, regional, and local resources) and sources of information for the interpretation of the occupational exposure profile also are included.

UNIT 2. OBTAINING AND INTERPRETING THE OCCUPATIONAL HISTORY

This unit concentrates on occupational history and on sources of information accessible to health professionals. It also discusses the selective use of occupational history, which can be obtained by a self-administered questionnaire before the face-to-face encounter with the health care provider begins. A suggested format for the screening occupational and environmental history is presented, with the comment that the use of a standard form is not a substitute for conscious attention to the oral interview.

The discussion includes reasons for obtaining the occupational history; levels of utilization of the occupational history (basic, diagnostic, screening, and comprehensive); and the structure and purpose of the occupational history form, in three parts: the occupational profile, the occupational exposure inventory, and the environmental history. Procedures in this unit address the use of the occupational history form to collect a data base, and integration of the occupational history with the clinical evaluation. In addition, the following are detailed: inventory of common hazardous exposures, inventory of occupations and corresponding major hazardous exposures, applications of the completed occupational history (patient evaluation, compensability, liability and risk control, screening, research, and community education), and factors which modify risk of occupationally related illness.

UNIT 3. CLINICAL ASSESSMENT OF THE OCCUPATIONAL CASE

Unit 3 discusses the acquisition of clinical data which may be brought to bear in a specific case. This is presented in the context of the preceding unit (i.e. the occupational history being a sensitive tool for the detection of possible occupational associations; a crude instrument when used alone for the detection of occupational illnesses).

This unit examines the application of the general medical interview, the physical examination, and laboratory and roentgenographic tests to cases of occupationally-related illness or injury. The approach is to show how these basic medical skills, in combination with the occupational history, provide a complete data base for clinical evaluation. Priority categories of occupational illness and injury are listed.

UNIT 4. EVALUATING THE OCCUPATIONALLY RELATED CASE

Unit 4 discusses the evaluation of an occupationally related case as a whole, applying all relevant information and focusing particularly on identifying occupational causes of disorders and their relationship to work. This unit examines the critical step of integrating findings from the occupational history and from the clinical assessment. The reader is guided in assessing the probable validity of the data obtained, integrating the data into a comprehensive evaluation of the case, and coming to a reasoned judgment on the questions of causation, occupational association, and disability.

The diagnosis is described as just the beginning of the evaluative process, the related but distinct questions of the causal exposure, the work-relatedness of the condition, and the expected degree of disability considered as important as a precise diagnosis. The concept of worker's compensation is addressed, explaining that the health care provider's conclusions about causation and work-relatedness have important implications within the worker's compensation system. A sample case report is included with the readings.

UNIT 5. PROVIDING OCCUPATIONAL HEALTH SERVICES

Unit 5 describes the procedures, services, and facilities functioning within the occupational health system, which affects all health care providers who see patients with work-related problems. It contrasts occupational cases with those within the practice of primary care as part of a much larger network of relationships that is formalized into this complex system. This unit also discusses the roles of primary care practitioners and occupational health professionals in this context.

UNIT 6. INTERVENTION STRATEGIES IN OCCUPATIONAL CASES

Unit 6 presents approaches to solving work-related health problems and ways to bring the resources of the occupational health system to bear for the benefit of the patient. It details means of correcting hazards in the workplace, from the point of view of the provider whose patient presents with an occupational disorder due to a hazard which continues to exist. An overview of the available technical approaches, usually used in combination to solve a particular occupational safety and health problem, is presented (eg, engineering controls, containment and inspection, personal protection, administrative controls, and behavioral controls).

This unit describes the role of the clinician with respect to corrective action. Two issues are mentioned: Without special training or expertise in occupational health, the provider is not technically qualified to recommend or advise on specific corrective measures and should concentrate on clearly stating the problem. Secondly, an insensitive or undiplomatic approach can cause great harm to the patient and may even cost the patient his/her job, regardless of the legal protection afforded the employee.

UNIT 7. STANDARDS IN OCCUPATIONAL HEALTH PRACTICE

This unit outlines standards in the provision of occupational health services (standards of practice, ethics, performance), whether practiced by the occupational health specialist, by the primary care provider who sees work-related disorders on an occasional basis, or by the specialist who performs consultations or special studies on a referral basis. It also presents an approach for evaluating how well these standards are attained.

The application of general health care standards to occupational health is described as particularly difficult and often challenging, as the provider in the occupational health care system is part of a much larger network which imposes its own constraints and balances the interests of the parties involved: the provider, the patient-employee, the employer, the workers' compensation carrier, the government (OSHA or its counterpart), and often, the employee's union. The one-to-one provider/patient relationship is modified into a hierarchy of responsibilities, which may be affected by law, government regulation, financial obligation, and obligations to the other parties.

REFERENCES

1. Segall AJ and Vanderschmidt HF (eds.): Health Maintenance in Clinical Practice. Boston: Boston University, Center for Educational Development in Health, 1985.

2. Doll R: Mortality from lung cancer in asbestos workers. Brit J Industrial Med 1955;12:81-86.

3. Doll R and Hill AB: Mortality in relationship to smoking: Ten years of observations of British doctors. Brit Med J 1964;I:1399-1410, 1460-1467.

4. Dawber TR: The Framingham Study: The Epidemiology of Atherosclerotic Disease. Cambridge, MA: Harvard University Press, 1980.

5. Multiple Risk Factor Intervention Trial (MRFIT) Research Group: Risk Factor Changes and Mortality Results. JAMA 1982;248(12):1465-1477.

6. Rose G, Hamilton PJS, Colwell L, Shipley MJ: A randomised controlled trial of anti-smoking advice: 10-year results. J Epidem Comm Health 1982;36:102-108.

7. Frame PS and Carlson SJ: A critical review of periodic health screening using specific screening criteria. J Fam Practice 1975; 2(1):29-36, 123-129, 189-194, 283-289.

8. Breslow L and Somers AR: The lifetime health monitoring program: A practical approach to preventive medicine. N Eng J Med 1977;296: 601-608.

9. Canadian Task Force on the Periodic Health Examination: The periodic health examination. Canad Med Assoc J 1979;121:1193-1254.

10. American Cancer Society: Guidelines for the cancer-related checkup: Recommendations and Rationale. CA - A Cancer Journal for Clinicians. American Cancer Society, 1980;30(4):194-240.

11. Farquhar JW: The American Way of Life Need Not be Hazardous to Your Health. New York: WW Norton, 1978.

12. American Heart Association: Coronary Risk Handbook. New York: American Heart Association, 1973.

13. Breslow L, et al: Risk Factor Update Project. Atlanta, GA: Centers for Disease Control, May 1982:235.

14. Goulding SA and Peterson PJ: Computerized health risk appraisal for adolescents. Health Educ 1983;14:34-35.

15. Maslow AH: Motivation and Personality (ed. 2). New York: Harper and Row, 1970.

16. McClelland D: The Achievement Motive (ed. 2). New York: Irvington Publishers, 1975.

Index

Accident prevention, 78-79

Adolescence and early adulthood, health behavior modification during, 42

Adolescent breast and testicular self-examinations, 84

Adolescent pregnancy prevention, 79-80

Age and hypertension, cardiovascular-renal abnormality and, 16-18

Anticipatory guidance, 72-73

Assessment
 health, see Health and risk assessment
 of potential learning problem in child, 69, 72

Behavior change, instructional units on motivating patient, 185
 referral for
  breast cancer, 198
  hypertension, 192
  primary care provider and, 187
 self-directed
  primary care provider and, 186-189
  smoking, 189

Behavior change programs
 goal setting in, 102-103, 112
 use of psychological testing for, 104-111
  in design of intervention program, 108-109
  in diagnosis, 108
  specific applications of, 110-111

Behavior problems in preventive health care, 94-95

Behavioral contracting, 104

Behavioral intervention, 93-117, 120-121
 and ambivalence toward behavioral change, 97
 control and
  locus of, 101-102
  losing, 97
 interventionist and
  appreciation according to temperament, 104
  propensities by temperament, 111
 role of, 95
 perceptual change as participant goal in, 102-103
 problem solving approaches to, 111-112
 responsibility assumption and, 95
  measuring, 101-102
 responsibility avoidance and, 96-97
 role of expectations in therapeutic alliance and, 99-101
 setting climate for, 98-99
 steps for, 97-98

Behavior intervention (Cont'd.)
techniques for
 behavioral rehearsal, 116-117
 creating internal commitment-
  setting goals, 112-113
 group program for eating modification, 120-121
 imagery rehearsal, 114-116
 relaxation training, 113-114

Behavioral outcomes and learning
 environments, 98-99

Behaviors, target vs. setting
 goals, 112

Blood pressure, high
 see Hypertension

Brazelton Neonatal Behavioral Scale
 (BNBAS), 69, 70-71

Breast cancer, instructional unit
 on, 197-199

Breast cancer mortality by age and
 five-year followup, 23

Breast self-examination (BSE),
 teenage, 84

Cardiovascular disease
 nutritional aspects of, instructional unit on, 193-196
 and obesity in young, 85
 value of epidemiology in, 16-19,
  20

Cardiovascular-renal abnormality
 and hypertension treatment, age
 and, 16-18

Cardiovascular risk factors in
 family practice center population, 25

Causal hypotheses, cohort and
 case-control studies and, 15

Causality, epidemiologic and
 related studies for, 14

Centers for Disease Control (CDC)
 questionnaire, 32, 49-50, 57-58

Child, healthy progress of, and
 family environment, 67

Children and adolescents, preventive initiatives for, see
 Pediatric practices

Clinical Health Maintenance:
 Guidebook, 183-201

Clinical prevention methods,
 29-44, 47-58
 comparison of sites for health
  maintenance services, 42-43
 development of health maintenance plan, 40
 health and risk assessment, 30,
  32-38, 39-40
 determination of health
  status, 32-34
 determination of risk status,
  34-38
 modification of health behavior
  during adolescence and early
  adulthood, 42
 risk status (health behavior)
  modification, 41-42
 selection of age-sex risk specific protocols, 39, 51-56

Clinical preventive medicine,
 definition, 48

Cognitive restructuring procedure,
 102-103

Cohort and case-control studies
 and causal hypotheses, 15
 instructional unit on, 178

Community oriented primary care
 (COPC) practice vs. usual primary care (PC) in hypertension
 control, 19, 20

Competency based training, value
 of, 157-158, 161

Computer-based information systems, 43
  to manage preventive initiative, 152, 153-154

Contract
  in pediatric practice, 63
  psychological
    behavioral contracting and, 104
    explicit vs. implicit, 100

Coronary artery disease, pediatric, early idenfication of risk factors and, 84-89

Coronary heart disease (CHD) mortality with special intervention (SI) vs. usual care (UC), 18-19, 20

Coronary risk factors, exercise training and, 85, 89

Costs in preventive initiatives, 139-148

Counseling and pediatric practice, 62

Death, causes of, 9, 35

Denver Depvelopmental Screening Test (DDST), 69

Determinants
  definition, 5
  of health, definition, 47
  of health status, 7, 9

Deterrents, definition, 5

Diabetes mellitus, screening for, 21-22

Diagnosis, true, screening-test results and, 21

Disease(s)
  acute infectious, 9-11
    epidemiology and prevention, 10

Disease(s) (Cont'd.)
  of adults, major asymptomatic remediable, 38
  chronic, natural history of, 12-13
  early identification of, in child, 80-83
  remediable and unrecognized, identification of risk factors and, 34-38

Distribution, definition, 5

Economic rewards for preventive activities, 3

Education
  in early childhood, for parents, 73
  health
    marketing vs., 89
    pediatric, 72-75
  sex, 79-80

Environmental exposure of children and youth, 75, 76
  home, 67

Epidemiologic and related studies for causality, 14

Epidemiologic basis of clinical prevention, 5-26
  acute infectious disease and, 9-11
  guidebook, 173, 175-179
  natural history of chronic disease and, 12-13
  risk factors and primary prevention, 14-16
  screening and secondary prevention, 19-24
    evaluating health impact of, 22-24
    tasks in adopting health maintenance plan, 24-26

Epidemiologic evidence, assessment of, instructional unit on, 176-178

Epidemiology
 defined, 5
 value of, in cardiovascular
  disease, 16-19,20

Epidemiology course results,
 evaluating, 164

Exercise training and coronary risk
 factors, 85, 89

Goal(s)
 behavioral change and, 102-103,
  112-113
 health, establishing, in young,
  63
 long-term preventive, 62
 objectives of teaching clinical
  prevention, 158, 161

Growth Charts, National Center of
 Health Statistics (NCHS), 67-68

Health
 defined, 7, 47
 by World Health Organization, 1
 and disease, McKeown model of, 36
 instructional unit on, 175

Health and risk assessment (HRA),
 30, 32-38 see also Health assessment
 definition, 48
 interpreting results of, instructional unit on, 185
 methods of, 39-40
  middle-aged adult, 53-54
  older adult, 55-56
  young adult, 51-52
 program sample, 57-58

Health and risk reassessment, definition, 48

Health assessment
 in pediatric practice, 64-72 see also Health and risk assessment
 purpose of, 30

Health assessment data, hypertension, instructional unit on, 190

Health behavior, definition, 47

Health behavior (risk status) modification, 41-42

Health care, behavior problems in
 preventive, 94-95

Health education
 marketing vs., 89
 pediatric, 72-75

"Health Fair", 74

Health habits, establishment of,
 in childhood, 62
 positive model and, 63-64

Health hazard, definition, 47

Health maintenance, definition, 47

Health maintenance agreement, definition, 48

Health maintenance examination,
 purposes of, 29

Health maintenance plan
 definition, 48
 development of, 40

Health maintenance services, comparison of sites for, 42-43

Health maintenance strategies in
 clinical practice, tasks required
 for, 24-26
 aids to implementation, 26
 practice population characteristics, 24-25
 state of the art alternatives, 24

Health promotion
 instructional units on, 175
 pediatric, 64-75
 smoking, and 188

Health promotion information,
  marketing of, 89

Health promotion visit in pediatric
  practices, 65, 66

Health protection, pediatrics,
  75-80

Health status
  definition, 48
  determinants, 7, 9
  determination of, 32-34
    objective assessment by health
      professional, 33-34
    subjective assessment by
      patient, 32-33
  instructional unit on, 175

Health status modification, definition, 48

Home Observation for Measurement of
  the Environment (HOME) inventory,
  67

Home Screening Questionnaire (HSQ),
  67

Hypertension
  instructional unit on, 190-192
  in pediatric population, 85
  treatment of, age and cardiovas-
    cular-renal abnormality and,
    16-18

Immunization
  instructional unit on, 196-197
  in pediatric practice, 75, 77-78
  schedule of, for normal infants
    and children, 77-78

Income from and costs associated
  with preventive initiatives, 3,
  139-148

Infants, health promotion visits
  for, 65, 66

Infectious disease
  child immunization and, 75
  epidemiology and, 9-11

Instructional series, annotated
  review of, 173-201
  guidebooks
    clinical health maintenance,
      183-201
    epidemiologic basis of clini-
      cal prevention, 173, 175-179
    management for preventive ser-
      vices, 179-183
  instructional units
    assessment of epidemiologic
      evidence, 176-178
    cancer of breast, 197-199
    health, 175
    hypertension, 190-192
    immunization, 196-197
    meeting population needs, 178-
      179
    nutritional aspects of car-
      diovascular disease, 193-196
    occupational health, 199-201
    risk and natural history of
      disease, 175-176
    smoking, 187-190
  overview of system, 173, 174

Instructional system, disseminating innovative, 170-171

Intervention, instructional units
  on
  direct, primary care provider
    and, 187
  monitoring and evaluating out-
    comes, 187
  selecting approach, 186
  selecting modality for smoking,
    188-189
  setting priorities, 186

Intervention techniques, behavioral, see Behavioral intervention techniques

Kellogg Project, 169-170

Kellogg Project's Dissemination
  Strategy, 170-171

Know Your Body (KYB) Program,
  73-74

Learning environments and behavioral outcomes, 98-99

Learning problem, assessment of potential, 69, 72

Management problems of practice in undertaking preventive initiatives, 122-154
  changes required, 123, 125-128
  developing income, 139-148
    identifying costs and risk, 141-148
    instructional unit on, 183
    third-party coverage, 140, 141
    total health care institutions, 140-141
  guidebook on, 179-183
  information systems, 148-153
  immunization, 197
    instructional units on, 183, 197
  kinds of practice, 122-123, 124-125, 133-134
  organization and objectives of medical practice, instructional unit on, 181
  organizing by developing protocols, 128-132
  smoking cessation as example
    identifying cost and risk, 144-148
    protocol flow chart, 131-132
    reasons for not placing patient in program, 131-132
    referral to outside resource, instructional unit on, 189
  staffing, 132-135
    instructional unit on, 182
  using community resources, 136-139
    evaluation of service, 138-139
    finding acceptable program, 137-139
    instructional units on, 182, 189
  smoking, 189
  using computers, 152, 153-154

Meyers Briggs Type Indicator (MBTI)
  description of, 105-107
  use of
    in designing intervention program, 108-109
    in diagnosis, 108
    specific applications, 110-111

Models
  classic, biomedical, 5-6
  expanding, medical, 7, 8
  McKeown, of health and disease, 36

Mortality, causes of
  untimely between ages of 1 and 65, 35
  in U.S., 1900-1980, 9

Multiple Risk Factor Intervention Trial (MRFIT), 16, 18
  decline in smoking among patients in (SI vs. UC), 134

Natural history of disease, instructional unit on, 176

Neurodevelopmental screening examination, 72

Nutritional aspects of cardiovascular disease, instructional unit on, 193-196

Nutritional guidance for young infant, 84

Obesity
  in adolescent female, 63
  and cardiovascular disease in young, 85

Occupational health, instructional unit on, 199-201

Pediatric population, hypertension in, 85

Pediatric practices, 58-59; see also Pediatric primary care, preventive initiatives in
  goals and approaches to primary prevention in, 60-64
    broad approach, 60, 62
    child's independence and participation, 63
    counseling, 62
    developmental stage, 60, 61
    dynamic growth and development of child, 62
    environment, 67
    establishing health goals, 63
    model of positive health habits, 63-64

Pediatric primary care, preventive initiatives in, 64-89
  assessment, 64-72
    parameters of growth, 67-68
    potential learning problem, 69, 72
  health education of parents, 72-75
  health promotion, 64-75
    anticipatory guidance, 72-73
    formats for visit, 65, 66
    high-risk infants, 65, 67
    self-care, 74
  health protection, 75-80
    accident prevention, 78-79
    identification of environmental hazards, 75, 76
    immunization, 75, 77-78
    teenage pregnancy prevention, 79-80
  prevention of illness, 80-89
    early identification of risk factors (example: coronary artery disease), 84-89
    hearing and vision problems, development and, 84
    obesity and cardiovascular disease, 85
    screening, 80-83

"Percent effectiveness", computing, 15-16

Pregnancy prevention, teenage, 79-80

Prenatal care, 65

Prevention
  in clinical medicine, definition, 47
  primary, 2, 14-16, 47
  secondary, 2, 19-24, 47

Preventive initiatives
  management problems of, see Management problems of practice in undertaking preventive initiatives

Preventive interventions, primary and secondary, 12

Preventive program evaluation, instructional unit on, 179

Preventive services, 51-56
  guidebook for implementing, 179-183
  for middle-aged adult, 53-54
  for older adult, 55-56
  for young adult, 51-52

Primary care
  community oriented (COPC) vs. usual (PC), hypertension control, 19, 20
  definition, 47
  pediatric, preventive initiatives in, 64-89

Primary prevention
  definition, 2, 47
  risk factors and, 14-16

Project Health PACT (Participatory and Assertive Consumer Training), 74-75

Protocols, developing, 128-132

Psychological testing in behavior change programs, 104-111

Relaxation training, 113-114

Risk
 absolute or relative or attributable, 14
 practice priorities and, 16-17
 assessing, see Health and risk assessment
 and environmental exposure in children and youth, 75, 76
 measuring, instructional unit on, 176
 and natural history of disease, instructional unit on, 175-176

Risk factor(s)
 anatomic and physiologic and biochemical, for adults, 37
 biologic and psychosocial, for infant, 65, 67
 definition, 47
 effect of multiple, on occurrence of cardiovascular disease, 17
 identification of, and remediable and unrecognized disease, 34-38
 primary prevention and, 14-16

Risk reduction, instructional unit on, 176

Risk specific protocols, selection of age-sex, 39, 51-56

Risk status
 definition, 48
 determination of, 34-38
 ability to cope with stress, 34
 identification of risk factors and remediable and unrecognized disease, 34-38
 initial screening for health and, instructional unit on, 185

Risk status modification, 41-42
 definition, 48

Rotter Internal/External Locus of Control Index, 101

Screening
 definition, 47
 for diabetes mellitus, 21-22
 evaluating health impact of, 22-24
 instructional unit on, 179
 for health and risk status, 185
 interpreting results, 187-188
 selecting packages and procedures, 185
 pediatric, 80-83
 for children and youth, 82-83
 for newborns, 81
 periodic multiphasic, 23
 secondary prevention and, 19-24

Screening test
 efficiency of, and predictive value positive (PVP), 21
 sensitivity and specificity of, 20-21

Secondary prevention, definition, 2, 47
 screening and, 19-24

Self-care
 instructional units on
 breast cancer, 198
 hypertension, 191
 pediatric, 74

Sex education, 79-80

Smoking
 instructional unit on, 187-190
 in MRFIT patients, decline in (SI vs. UC), 134

Smoking cessation initiative
 income analysis of, 144-148
 information system for, 149-153
 practice-staffed, 134-135

Smoking cessation programs, checklist to evaluate, 139

Smoking cessation protocol flow chart, 131-132

Stress, ability to cope with, 34

"Teachable moment"
  for child, 73
  definition, 41

Teaching, didactic, vs. active
  learning, 162

Teaching of preventive medicine,
156-172
  active learning and, 162, 169
  evaluation of results of, 164-169
    performance checklist, 166-167
    performance testing mechanism,
      advantage and disadvantage
      of, 165
  goals and objectives of, 158, 161
  model teaching sites for, 170
  patient flow patterns, 162, 163
    how to design, instructional
      unit on, 181-182
  planning courses for, 161-164
  and scarcity and poor quality of
  courses in prevention, 156-158
    performance analysis of prac-
      ticing physicians and nurses,
      169
  student attitudes, questionnaires
    gauging, 164, 168
  target population of, 161
  value of competency based
    training in, 157-158, 161
  vertical and horizontal integra-
    tion in, 158, 159-160

Testicular self-examination (TSE),
  adolescent, 84

World Health Organization definition of health, 1